WATERSIDE WALKS
in Cumbria &
the Lake District

Mark S. Elliott

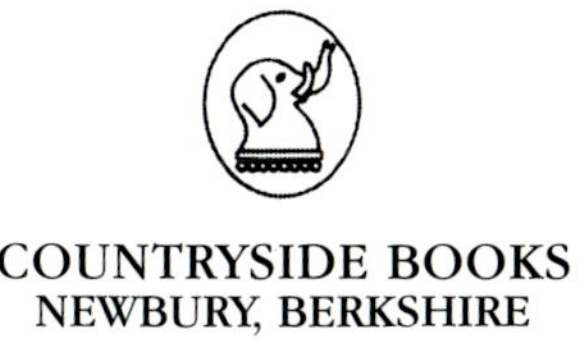

COUNTRYSIDE BOOKS
NEWBURY, BERKSHIRE

COUNTRYSIDE BOOKS
3 Catherine Road
Newbury, Berkshire

To view our complete range of books,
please visit us at
www.countrysidebooks.co.uk

ISBN 978 1 84674 135 7

In memory of Norman Hewson, 'Gramps'

Cover picture of Rydal Water
supplied by David Sellman

Maps by Gelder Design & Mapping
Photographs by the author

Designed by Peter Davies, Nautilus Design
Produced through MRM Associates Ltd., Reading
Typeset by Jean Cussons Typesetting, Diss, Norfolk
Printed in Thailand

Contents

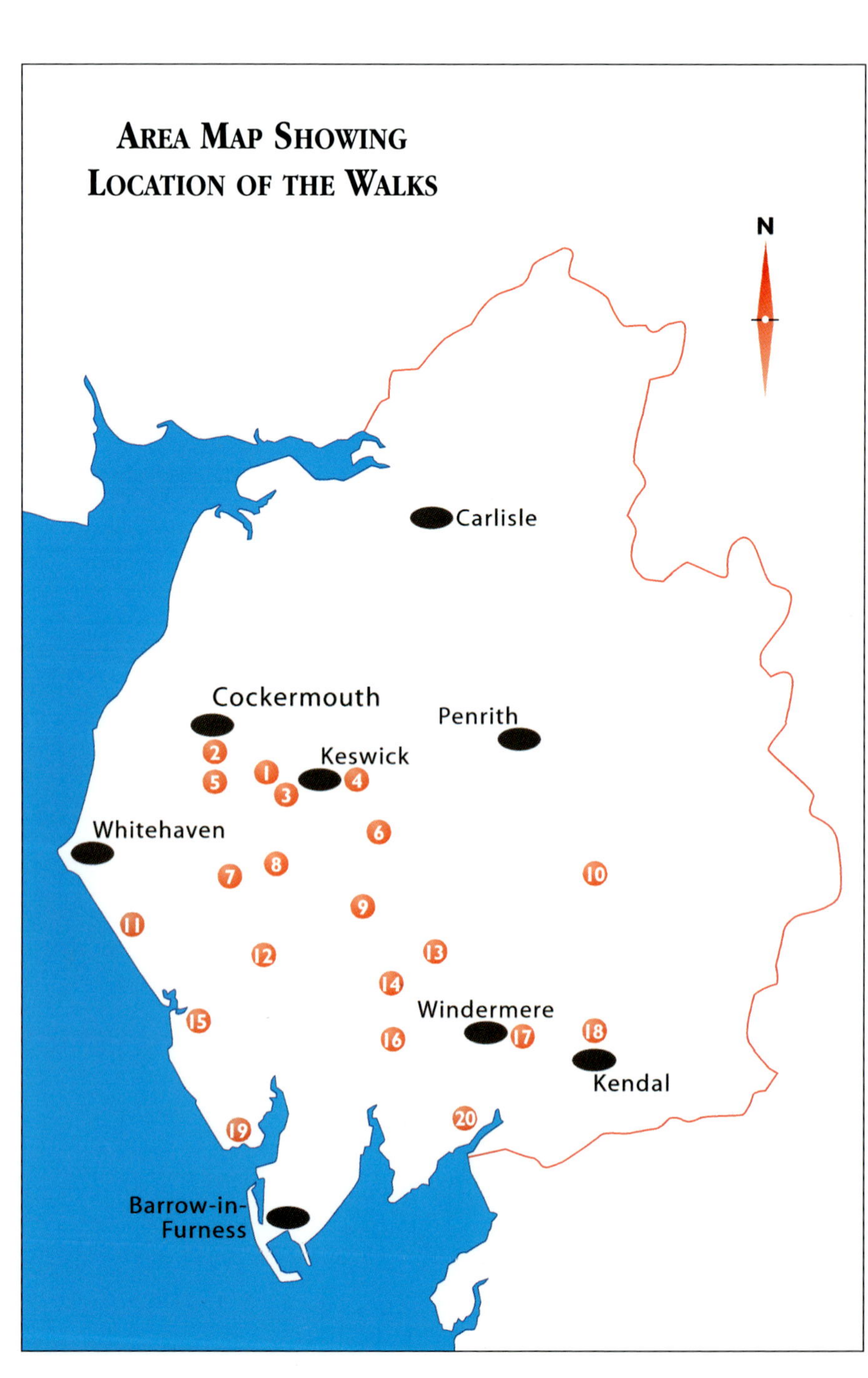

Area Map Showing
Location of the Walks
N
Carlisle
Cockermouth
Penrith
Keswick
Whitehaven
Windermere
Kendal
Barrow-in-Furness

PUBLISHER'S NOTE

We hope that you obtain considerable enjoyment from this book; great care has been taken in its preparation. Although at the time of publication all routes followed public rights of way or permitted paths, diversion orders can be made and permissions withdrawn.

We cannot, of course, be held responsible for such diversion orders and any inaccuracies in the text which result from these or any other changes to the routes nor any damage which might result from walkers trespassing on private property. We are anxious though that all details covering the walks are kept up to date and would therefore welcome information from readers which would be relevant to future editions.

The simple sketch maps that accompany the walks in this book are based on notes made by the author whilst checking out the routes on the ground. They are designed to show you how to reach the start, to point out the main features of the overall circuit and they contain a progression of numbers that relate to the paragraphs of the text.

However, for the benefit of a proper map, we do recommend that you purchase the relevant Ordnance Survey sheet covering your walk. The Ordnance Survey maps are widely available, especially through booksellers and local newsagents.

INTRODUCTION

Each year, millions of visitors flood into Cumbria, attracted by its magnificent scenery. The Lake District is the jewel in Cumbria's crown. Its rugged peaks and shimmering lakes entice outdoor enthusiasts, photographers and painters, as well as those who simply want to admire the wonderful views.

The Lakeland summits attract walkers who like a challenge and the reward of stunning panoramas. But there is much more to Cumbria than its Lake District, and more to the Lake District than its mountain summits. The Cumbrian coastline and valleys offer gentler terrain,

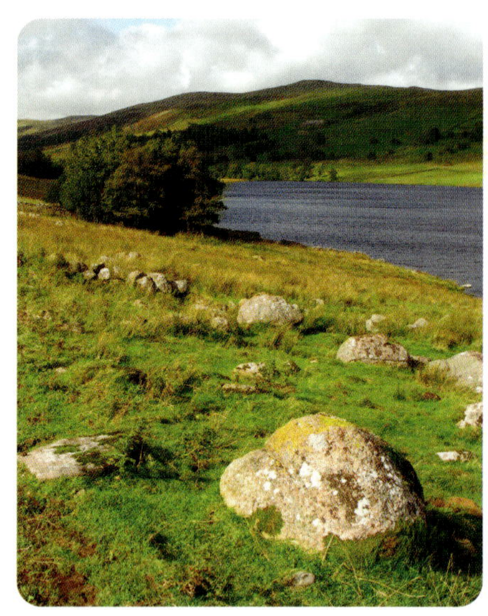

Sleddale Reservoir

which is beautiful and rich in flora and fauna. These areas have fascinating histories and traces of their past often remain – perfect for walkers looking for something less strenuous and more interesting than mountain-bagging.

This book contains twenty walks which share a common theme: they all pass beside picturesque waterside locations. In most cases, the going is easy and little climbing is involved. A description of the walk and the terrain is given at the start of each walk. A simple map is also provided. This is only a guide, and I strongly recommend that you also carry an Ordnance Survey map of the area in which you intend to walk. You should also be properly equipped for the outdoors, with suitable footwear and clothing and remember to take extra care when walking along roads without pavements.

I have thoroughly enjoyed researching all the walks for this book and have discovered many new places and fascinating facts along the way. I hope you enjoy the book and have many happy days in the Cumbrian countryside.

Mark S. Elliott

NEWLANDS BECK FROM BRAITHWAITE

This journey takes you from Braithwaite, with its jumble of old buildings, up onto the flanks of Barrow Fell, which rises above the village. There are lovely views across the Newlands Valley towards the popular peak of Cat Bells. You return through farmland alongside the clear waters of Newlands Beck, with views across to Skiddaw.

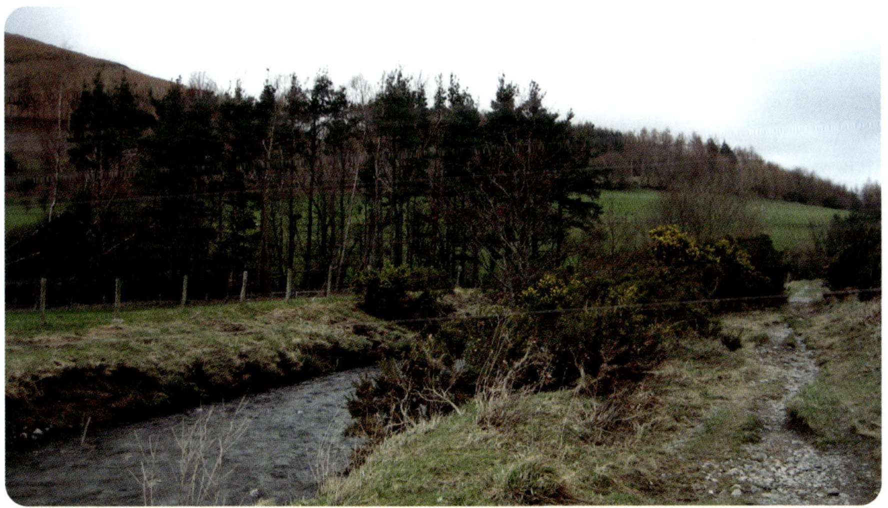

The footpath beside Newlands Beck

- **HOW TO GET THERE:** From Keswick follow the A66 and then follow the B5292 into Braithwaite. Turn right before the Royal Oak pub. St Herbert's church is on the right.
- **PARKING:** Limited roadside parking is available near Braithwaite school, a short distance from the church.
- **LENGTH OF THE WALK:** 3.8 miles/6.2 kilometres. **MAP:** OS Explorer OL4 (GR NY 232237).
- **TERRAIN:** Mostly easy going along obvious paths, with one uphill section. Numerous stiles along the route make it very difficult to take along all but the smallest of dogs.

Braithwaite lies at the foot of Whinlatter Pass, beside Coledale Beck. The name Braithwaite is believed to have originated from Old Scandinavian *breiðr þveit* 'broad clearing'. The village grew to support the local woollen and lead mining industries that flourished here. The oldest parts of the village are a jumble of stone buildings close to the Royal Oak pub, which itself dates back over 200 years.

Your walk starts from St Herbert's church, which was built in 1900 as a chapel of ease. The route picks its way through the village and then crosses Coledale Beck. A short, easy climb takes you past Braithwaite Lodge Farm and then onto the flanks of Barrow Fell. The fell was extensively mined for lead in the past. Barrow mine opened in the 17th century and eventually closed in 1888. The old spoil heaps can still be seen sweeping down to the road.

Your route then descends gradually, passing Uzzicar Farm, which dates from the 16th century. The name Uzzicar originates from the wide, shallow lake called Husaker Tarn, which was once located here. It was drained in the 13th century by the monks of Furness Abbey to make new land for cultivation; hence the area became known as the Newlands Valley.

The return leg follows the river bank along the pretty Newlands Beck. Its clear water bubbles over a rocky riverbed towards Lake Bassenthwaite. Look out for kingfishers. The final part of your walk joins Coledale Beck and follows its bank back into the village of Braithwaite, where you can stop off at the Royal Oak to sample some of their excellent Jennings beers and hearty food, telephone: 01768 778533.

THE WALK

1. From the church head towards the Royal Oak. At the road junction in front of the pub, turn right and then immediately left, passing down the road at the back of the pub. Continue over the small road bridge which crosses the Coledale Beck. Follow the road, passing the corner shop on your right. You now pass several houses. As you go past the last house on the right, look for a farm track which climbs the hillside towards Braithwaite Lodge Farm. Turn right here and climb the track towards the farm. Go through the farmyard until you reach a four-way wooden fingerpost. Keep straight on for a short distance, following the Newlands sign.

2. Shortly after passing a stone wall you will reach a junction in the path. Ignore the path that climbs up the steep section of fellside, towards the

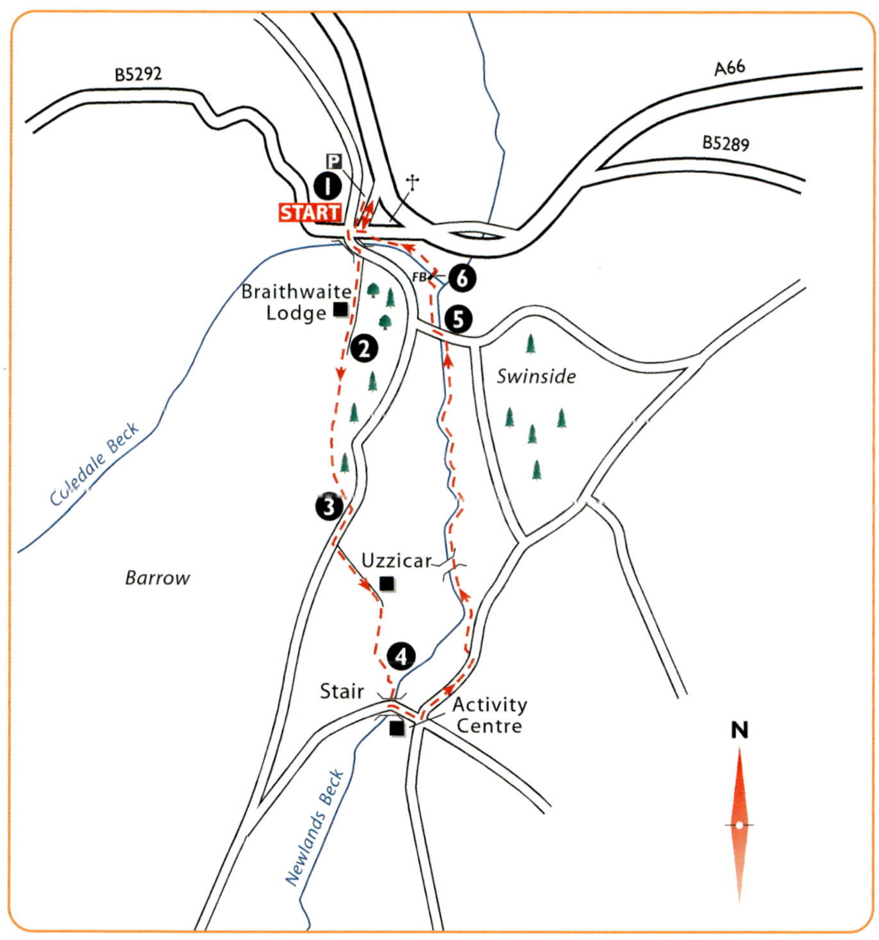

summit of Barrow. Instead, bear left and follow the path that skirts the top of the wood, which contains silver birch trees. The route then traverses the bracken-covered fellside, passing Scots pines before descending towards the road. In front of you are good views up the Newlands valley.

3. Turn right when you reach the road. Continue along the road. On your right you will see expanses of spoil from the old mine workings. Carry on until you reach the entrance to Uzzicar Farm. Turn left here and follow the public footpath that leads towards the farm. Bear right immediately before reaching the farm and continue along a rough track.

Cross the wooden step-stile beside the gate and continue ahead. Follow the footpath markers through the farm field, keeping generally to the right and following the fence line. Cross another step-stile and continue as before.

4. Turn right when you reach a farm track. This leads you towards a stone road bridge that crosses Newlands Beck. The hamlet here is called Stair. Go through the metal gate onto the road, and then turn left to cross the bridge. Newlands Adventure Centre is on your right. Continue down the road, ignoring the minor road on your right. Carry on until you see a wooden fingerpost on your left which directs you along the river bank back towards Braithwaite. Follow the river bank footpath over a series of stiles. You will pass beside an old packhorse bridge along the trail.

5. You will reach a wooden gate that leads onto a road next to a road bridge over the beck. Go left here, over the bridge, and head towards the nearby farm. Turn right here. Follow the wooden fingerpost for Braithwaite that leads you towards the farmyard, and then follow the short permissive path which diverts you around the farmyard. Pass through a wooden gate and then rejoin the river bank. Follow the beck, go through another wooden gate, and then continue along the river bank path.

6. The path bends to the left, leaving the Newlands Beck river bank and joins the bank of its tributary, Coledale Beck. Look for a wooden footbridge on your right, which crosses Coledale Beck. Cross over the bridge and then turn left. You will see a caravan park ahead of you. Carry on, crossing a wooden stile, and continue along the edge of the caravan park. Follow the path beside the river, which takes you behind rows of caravans. Proceed down a short section of path which leads you between the river and some houses. You will emerge onto a road in front of a stone building. Turn left here, and then follow the road a short distance to the junction. Turn right to retrace your steps through the village, towards the Royal Oak and your starting point.

NEARBY ATTRACTION
Whinlatter Visitor Centre at the top of Whinlatter Pass (B5292). The centre includes a café, woodland trails, mountain bike routes and a high-wire course.

RIVER COCKER FROM COCKERMOUTH

This is an easy ramble through farmland along the banks of the enchanting River Cocker. The route passes three former mills, evidence of the important role that the river played in powering 17th- and 18th-century industry.

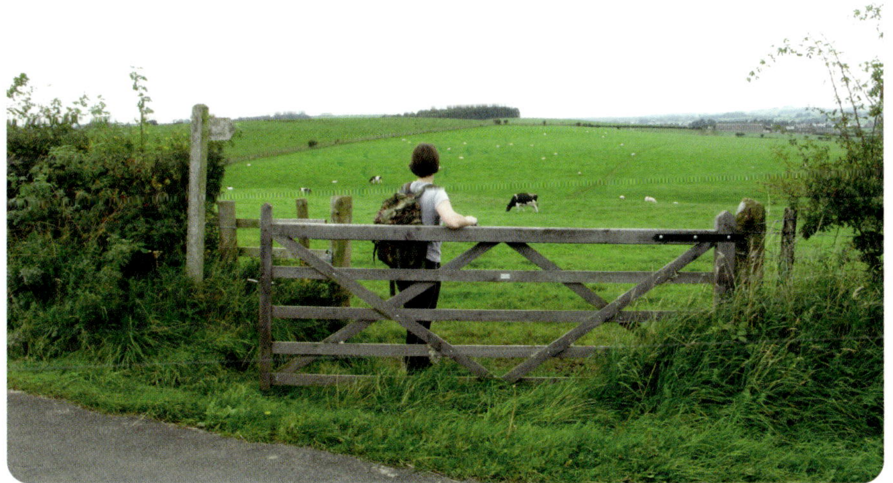

Heading off onto the farmland

- **HOW TO GET THERE:** From Keswick follow the A66 west for approximately 12 miles. You will reach a large roundabout next to the Sheep and Wool Centre. Take the third exit and continue towards Cockermouth. When you reach a set of traffic lights, bear right, and then turn left at the mini-roundabout into Sainsbury's.
- **PARKING:** Large pay-and-display car park next to Sainsbury's.
- **LENGTH OF WALK:** 4.9 miles/7.8 kilometres. **MAP:** OS Explorer OL4 and 303 (GR NY 120304).
- **TERRAIN:** Mostly flat and occasionally muddy farm fields. The route crosses farmland, and livestock are often present. There are numerous stiles along the route, which makes taking along all but the smallest of dogs very difficult.

Your walk starts from Cockermouth, a fabulous little West Cumbrian town, best known as the birthplace of William Wordsworth, in April 1770. The impressive Georgian house where he was born stands on Main Street and is open to the public. Fletcher Christian, of *Mutiny on the Bounty* fame, also has strong links to the town. He was born at Moorland Close, near Cockermouth, in 1764, and was schooled at Cockermouth Free Grammar School.

The name *Cocker* is of Celtic origin and means 'crooked'. The river flows out of Crummock Water and winds its crooked way down the Lorton Valley before reaching the town of Cockermouth, which derives its name from its location at the mouth of the river. The mouth of the River Cocker is not on the coast but at the place where it joins the River Derwent, which ultimately reaches the sea at Workington.

The first part of your walk, along the tree-lined passageway beside the Fire HQ, follows the course of the old Cockermouth and Workington railway line, which was built in 1865. Cockermouth station stood on what is now the site of the Fire HQ. The station opened to passenger traffic on 2nd January 1865, and closed on 18th April 1966.

The route continues beside the River Cocker and passes near Double Mills Youth Hostel. The building was originally a 17th-century watermill, although it is believed that a mill has stood on this site since the 1400s. This mill was known as a 'double' mill because it had two waterwheels operating two separate sets of gearing and millstones. The old waterwheels can still be seen to the left of the entrance. The mill was disused by 1900, bought by the urban district council in 1902, and was let to the YHA in 1933.

THE WALK

1. Leave Sainsbury's car park by the exit located opposite the petrol station. Turn right and then cross over the road. Follow the pavement as it bends to the left in front of the war memorial. This leads you down a passageway between two fences. Over the fence on your right is the Fire HQ. Continue down the tree-lined passage until you reach the concrete walls of the bridge over the River Cocker.

2. Immediately after crossing the bridge, turn right to follow the greenway sign displaying a yellow badge inscribed 'public footpath, Double Mills, Southwaite'. This path runs through a wooded area, roughly parallel to the river on your right. Continue along this path, ignoring the left turning which ascends a series of steps. The path

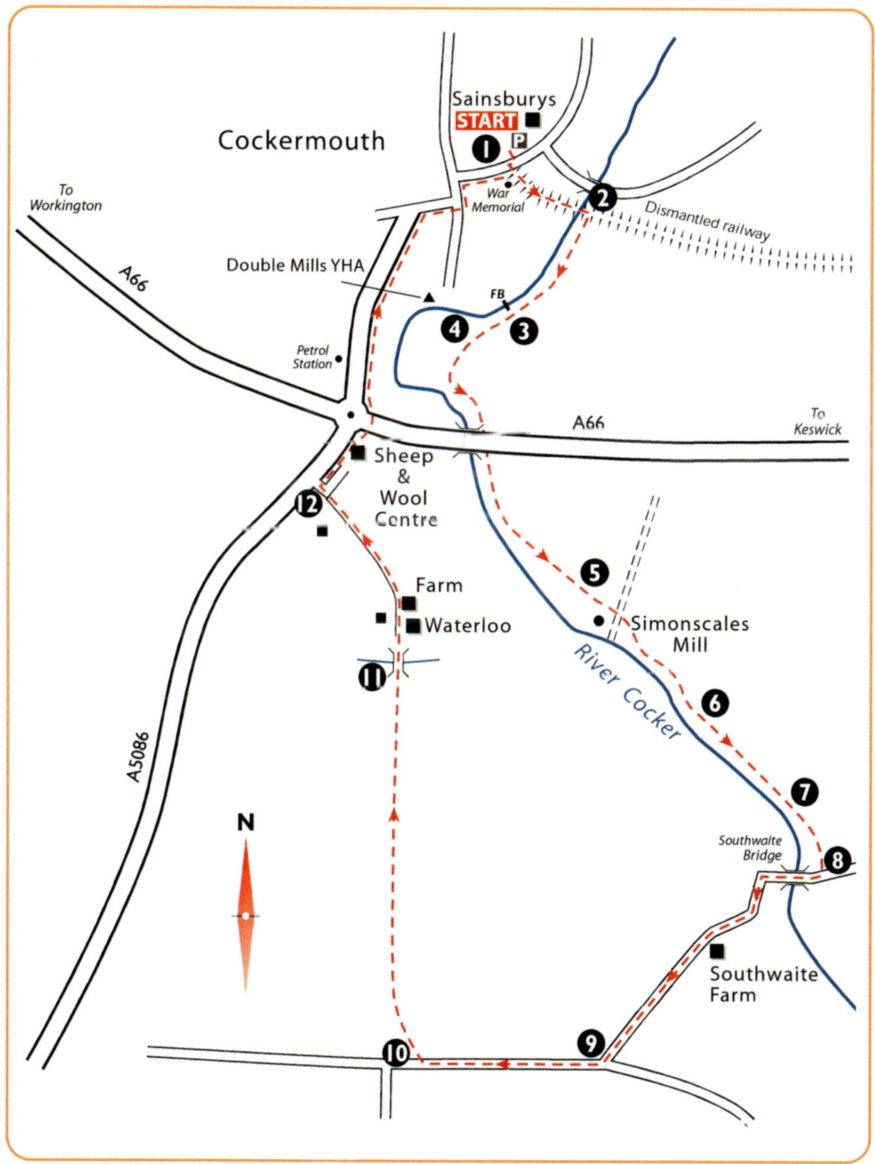

crosses a small low wooden footbridge and then enters a field. Continue along the edge of the field beside a line of trees. A children's play area is located over to your left. Proceed until you reach Double Mills footbridge, which spans the river.

3. Go straight on, passing the footbridge on your right, and through the kissing gate ahead of you. The path now follows the river bank for a short section. On the opposite side of the river you will see Double Mills Youth Hostel.

4. Cross the field ahead of you and then rejoin the river bank. Bear left and follow the river bank path, with the river on your right. Continue over a stile and go under the A66 road bridge. The path continues along the edge of the field. Cross another step stile and continue to walk beside the river. The path now crosses a meadow and then continues past Simonscales Mill Cottages, formerly a paper mill which developed during the mid 18th-century boom in demand for paper.

5. A wooden step stile with an attached fingerpost leads you onto a farm track. Cross over this track and then go over the next stile and into another field. Continue through the fields, with the river on your right. Cross a small low wooden footbridge over a tiny stream and proceed through the next field.

6. Cross two stiles with a boggy section between them. Carry on through another field, where a rusty old bath beside the fence acts as a cattle trough. Follow the faint path beside a fence line.

7. Look out for two footpath badges on the fence. Bear right just after them and descend through a narrow muddy path towards the river. Climb a step stile into a small lush field. Pass under some power lines and then go over another step stile. Follow the lower path, which keeps close to the river. Descend several wooden steps and drop down to another small meadow. An attractive stone bridge comes into view ahead of you. Walk beside the river for a short distance, and then bear left to go over a wooden step stile next to a metal gate. This takes you onto the road.

8. Once on the road, turn right and cross over the bridge. This is Southwaite Bridge and was constructed in 1890. Carry on past another converted mill – Southwaite Mill Cottages. An old millstone can be seen in front of the building on your left. Follow the road.

9. When you reach the sweeping right-hand bend in the road, bear right, following the roadside sign for Eaglesfield. Continue along the country lane, passing an attractive detached house on your left and the entrance to Low Hall.

10. Carry on along the road until you see a wooden fingerpost marked 'public bridleway', on your right. At this point bear right, leaving the road through a wooden gate and continuing into a large open field. Keep straight ahead, passing through the centre of the field towards the buildings you can see in the distance. The path is faint. At the far side of the field go through a large wooden gate which displays a public bridleway badge. Keep going straight ahead towards a large grey barn.

11. Cross a small stream by means of a small, wooden, sleeper bridge, and then cross a stile next to a metal gate. Continue straight on along a section of farm track with hawthorn hedges on each side. Pass the large grey barn on your right and then go through a metal gate beside a smaller, corrugated barn. You will pass a small farm on your right. Keep straight ahead, through a set of double metal gates and along a concrete track. You will then emerge onto the road which leads into the Shepherds' Hotel and Visitor Centre (a sheep and wool centre). Bear slightly left and head towards the main road (A5086), which is in front of you.

12. Turn right when you reach the main road and proceed towards a large roundabout. At the roundabout, cross over the A66 and keep straight on, towards Cockermouth, passing a petrol station on your left. Follow the road, which climbs gradually and then descends towards the town. When you reach the traffic lights bear right towards your starting point.

NEARBY ATTRACTIONS

Wordsworth House, the birth place of William Wordsworth, is located on Cockermouth's Main Street and is open to the public. Cockermouth has an excellent selection of galleries, coffee shops, cafés, pubs and restaurants. **Jennings Brewery** runs brewery tours in the afternoons on most days. Tourist information is available at Cockermouth Tourist Information Centre, Town Hall, Market St, Cockermouth, CA13 9NP, telephone: 01900 822634.

DERWENTWATER FROM PORTINSCALE

This walk passes the gates of Lingholm, where Beatrix Potter spent many of her summer holidays and where she found inspiration for several of her books. The trail follows the shoreline of Derwentwater through attractive woodland at Brandelhow. It is mostly flat and follows easy paths, culminating with an enjoyable boat trip back to Nichol End, near the start of your walk.

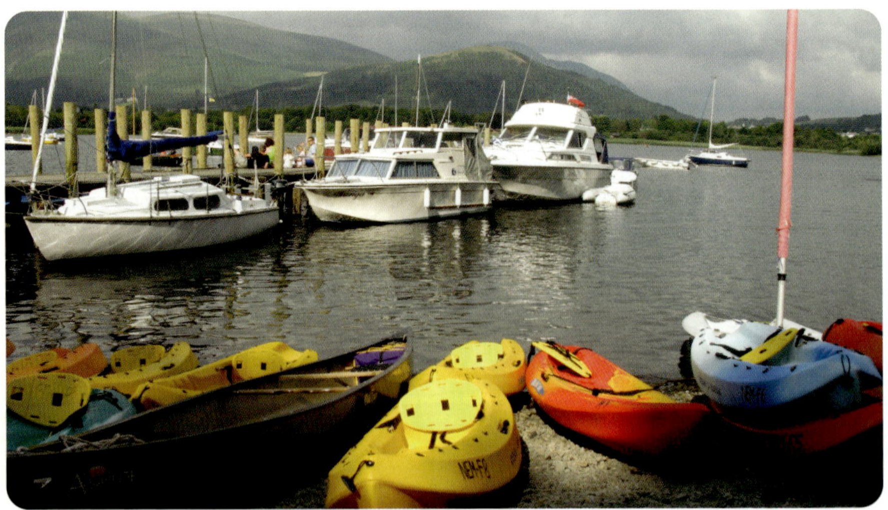

Nichol End

- **HOW TO GET THERE:** The village of Portinscale is located just over a mile west of Keswick. Take the A66 west and then exit at the sign for Portinscale. Continue through the village and then turn left at a junction on a sweeping right-hand bend. The Derwentwater Hotel is on the right and the small suspension bridge is at the bottom of this road.
- **PARKING:** Limited roadside parking is available near the suspension bridge just beyond the hotel.
- **LENGTH OF WALK:** 6.2 miles/9.9 kilometres. **MAP:** OS Explorer OL4 (GR NY 253237).
- **TERRAIN:** Mostly level, easy terrain with obvious paths.

Your walk starts from the village of Portinscale, situated just over a mile from Keswick. Neolithic man lived here, and four ancient stone axes and other artefacts were uncovered in the village in 1901. The site is believed to have been where axes were finished, or polished.

Your route passes Nichol End, which provides boat moorings and is the location of a jetty for the popular Keswick passenger launch. In days gone by, pilgrims used this point to cross the lake to the nearby island, which was the home of St Herbert, a 7th-century monk. In the 14th century, a shrine was erected to St Nicholas, the patron saint of sailors, where pilgrims prayed for their safety before crossing the lake. The area became known as St Nicholas's landing and later as Nichol End.

You will pass the gates of Lingholm, where, between 1885 and 1907, Beatrix Potter spent nine summer holidays. The garden and surrounding area provided inspiration for many of her books; the vegetable garden at Lingholm, with its wicket gate, can be seen in *The Tale of Peter Rabbit*.

Your route continues through the woodland at Brandelhow, which in 1902 was one of the National Trust's first purchases. The opening ceremony was performed by HRH Princess Louise, a daughter of Queen Victoria, on 6 October 1902. En route a beautifully carved pair of wooden hands can be seen, that celebrate the centenary of the purchase.

The last part of your journey crosses the lake by passenger launch, returning you to Nichol End. It is an opportunity to relax for a while and take in the beauty of the lake and the fabulous scenery which surrounds it.

THE WALK

Note: Ensure that you give yourself plenty of time to reach the jetty point in time to board the last motor launch. Check the timetables for departure times.

1. From the Derwentwater Hotel in Portinscale, follow the road into the centre of the village. Turn left at the T-junction on the sweeping bend in the road, following the sign for 'Launches, Nichol End and Derwentwater Marina'. Pass the tea rooms and gift shop on your right and continue along the road, passing Derwentwater Marina.

2. Follow the roadside pavement until you reach the turning for Nichol End Marina (signed). Turn left here and leave the road. Follow the side track towards Nichol End. Just before you reach the shop, go right and pass beside a wooden gate.

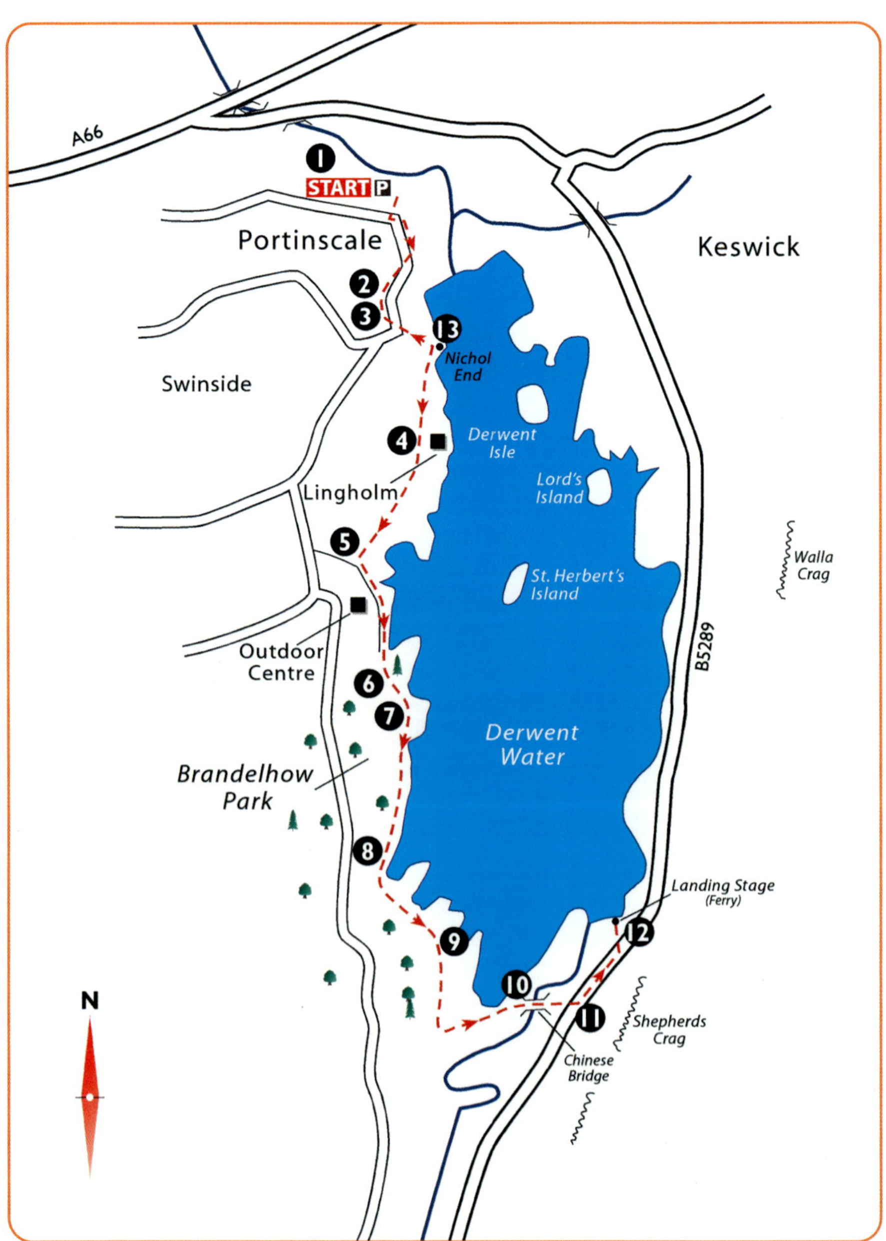

3. Once through the gate, the path ascends to reach a tarmac road with a stone house on the left. Cross over this road and continue down the track directly opposite the house. The track passes through woodland fringed with rhododendrons.

4. Emerge at the entrance to Lingholm. To the right of the entrance, go through the kissing gate marked 'public footpath to Cat Bells'. Follow the track through shaded woodland, with Scots pines on your right. You will reach a wooden kissing gate which leads you into an open meadow dotted with trees. You will see Cat Bells ahead of you. If you look closely you might see walkers toiling up its ridge. Continue along the obvious path to a gate on a small wooden bridge. Your route then climbs up into more woodland.

5. You will reach another kissing gate and a tarmac road at a minor junction. Take the second turning on your left, following the tarmac road. After a short distance you will reach the Hawes End Centre. Follow the road as it sweeps left in front of the centre. A metal fence then lines the edge of the road.

6. After a few minutes' walk you will see a metal gate and a kissing gate on your left. Turn left here, leaving the road, and descend through a sloping field towards the lake. You will pass an unusual bench on your left, which has been carved out of a tree trunk. Derwentwater is visible on your left.

7. Continue down the obvious path, passing through another two gates, until you reach the lake and a small jetty. Go right here, through a kissing gate, and into Brandelhow Woods, keeping the lake to your left. You will soon reach a beautifully-carved pair of wooden hands, which celebrate 100 years of The National Trust. Continue to follow the woodland track.

8. When you reach Brandelhow jetty, the path carries on ahead, but a pleasant diversion goes left here to follow the water's edge around Brandlehow Bay. An attractive boathouse is visible on the other side of the bay. Arrive at a house called Brandelhow and continue through a kissing gate and down the track, passing Rupert's Wood on your right. Pass the entrance to Abbot's Bay House and continue along a section of tarmac road until, on your right, you reach a single storey house called The Warren. Turn left immediately opposite this house, leaving the road and following the track into mature woodland.

9. Continue past Myrtle Bay. Stick to the main path and carry on until you reach a gate through a stone wall. Pass through this and emerge from the woods into an open area. Ahead of you are views towards the Borrowdale valley. Tree-covered Castle Crag is visible in the middle distance. Continue along the boardwalk section as it crosses the boggy ground at the southern end of the lake. Orchids grow in this area.

10. Go over the attractive bridge, known as the Chinese Bridge, that crosses the River Derwent. This is a nice spot for a rest and a chance to watch trout, that are often visible under the bridge, and the rock climbers on Shepherds Crag opposite.

11. Continue until you reach a stone wall with a stone stile over it. Climb over the stile, onto the roadside (B5289). Turn left and follow the pavement, passing the Lodore Falls Hotel on your right. Soon after passing the hotel you will reach a metal gate and a kissing gate on your left. A sign reads 'Keswick launch'. Go through the gate and head towards the lake and jetty.

12. Take the passenger launch from the jetty to Nichol End. The launch that travels round the lake in a *clockwise* direction will reach your destination soonest; another passenger launch travels in an anti-clockwise direction around the lake, and requires you to leave the boat at the Keswick terminus and then join another boat, which travels to Nichol End.

13. After arriving at Nichol End, retrace your route to Portinscale. Refreshments are available from the café at Nichol End and the tea rooms in Portinscale.

NEARBY ATTRACTION
Keswick is a popular tourist town with a wide variety of pubs, cafés, restaurants and other attractions. More information can be obtained from Keswick Tourist Information Centre, Moot Hall, Keswick, Cumbria, CA12 5JR, telephone: 017687 72645.

THE RIVER GRETA FROM KESWICK

This walk is a delightful blend of beautiful countryside and industrial heritage. Splendid woodland paths and the remnants of a Victorian railway track combine to make this a ramble to remember. The impressive River Greta is your companion throughout; it occasionally disappears out of sight but is never far away.

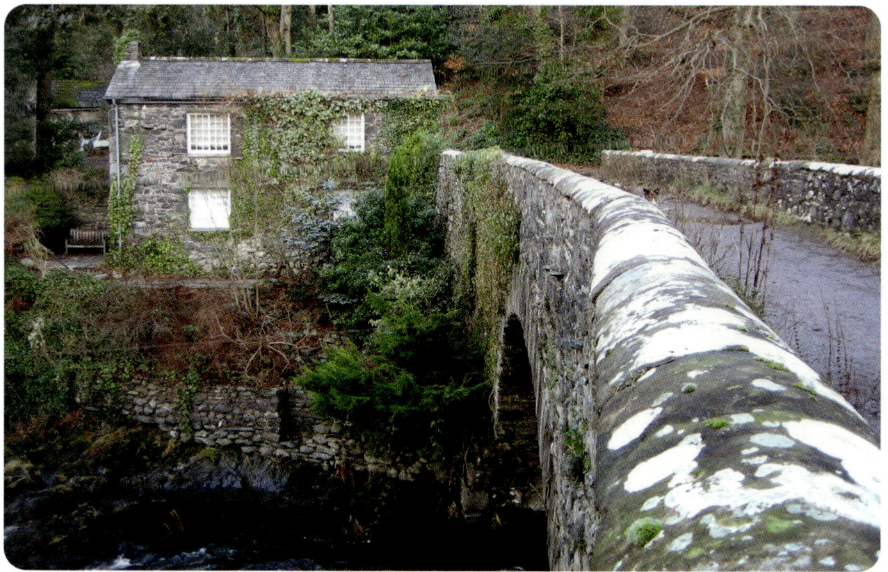

Old Greta Bridge

- **HOW TO GET THERE:** Keswick is located in the northern Lake District, just off the A66. The Keswick Pool and Fitness Centre is located on Station Road, just past Keswick Museum and Gallery (signed).
- **PARKING:** Limited free parking is available just off Brundholme Road and on Station Road.
- **LENGTH OF WALK:** 3.9 miles/6.3 kilometres. **MAP:** OS Explorer OL4 (GR NY 270237).
- **TERRAIN:** An easy route along obvious paths; some undulating sections through the woodland.

The first part of your walk leaves Keswick, the popular Lake District tourist town, and heads in the general direction of Penrith. You venture into Brundholme Woods, which is mixed woodland that is rich in wildlife. Keep an eye out for the roe deer, red squirrels and woodpeckers that live here. You might find wild strawberries or raspberries growing along your route in late summer.

An undulating path picks its way through the woods. The going is generally easy, with a few short sections that require you to be more energetic.

The River Greta is recognized and protected as a Special Area of Conservation (SAC) and a Site of Special Scientific Interest (SSSI), and conservation efforts have been rewarded with the return of otters to the area. The river is popular with anglers, who can often be seen stalking its brown trout, sea trout and salmon. Canoeists also regularly test themselves against the river's rapids.

The return leg follows the course of the old Cockermouth, Keswick and Penrith railway line and illuminates the area's fascinating industrial heritage. On the last part of your ramble, several of the area's famous peaks come into view: Cat Bells, Causey Pike and Skiddaw. Your journey ends at the old Keswick railway station – a final reminder of days gone by and a wonderful walk.

THE WALK

1. From the Keswick Pool and Fitness Centre, head towards Keswick town centre. Take the gate into Fitz Park, located on your left, opposite Keswick Museum. Keep right, following the path towards the river. Cross the River Greta at the new footbridge. Turn left here and follow the A5271 out of Keswick. This section of the walk follows the road for half a mile, but you will soon escape into countryside. You can avoid walking along the pavement for a short distance by cutting through an iron gate opposite the Millfield retirement home and following the riverbank path. Rejoin the pavement just before the iron railway bridge crosses overhead. Continue following the road, passing Townsfield on your left. Soon afterwards, leave the main road and travel down Forge Lane, which branches to your left.

2. Continue down Forge Lane to a small hamlet. Watch for a left turning, which you need to take to cross the river by means of a picturesque stone bridge. Once over the bridge, turn immediately right through a kissing gate and enter Brundholme Wood. Follow the rising path as it

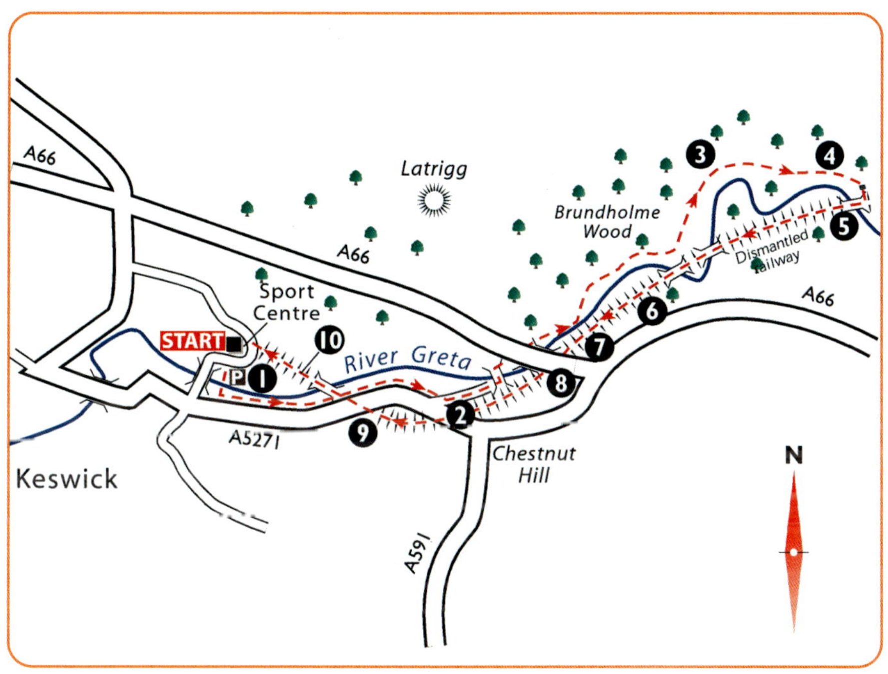

passes under the concrete bridge which carries the A66 over the valley. The path is a little steep at this point. In late summer you can find wild strawberries on the bank to your left.

3. Keep to the woodland path. Good views of the river start to unfold as you pass through mixed woodland of oak, birch, beech and conifers. You might catch a glimpse of roe deer and red squirrels. Ignore any minor paths that branch from the main path. Look out for a superb view of a horseshoe bend in the river, which you can admire from a high point along the trail.

4. On your right-hand side, keep an eye out for a major path which descends towards the river in a series of steps. Take this path, The track leads you to the edge of the river. In front of you are a succession of rapids and a deep pool, and heron are frequently seen fishing here. Follow the path upstream as it skirts the riverbank. Continue until you reach a stile into an open field. In the distance ahead of you are the flanks of Blease Fell. Cross the stile, and then immediately bear right and descend into the lower field. You will now see the route of the old

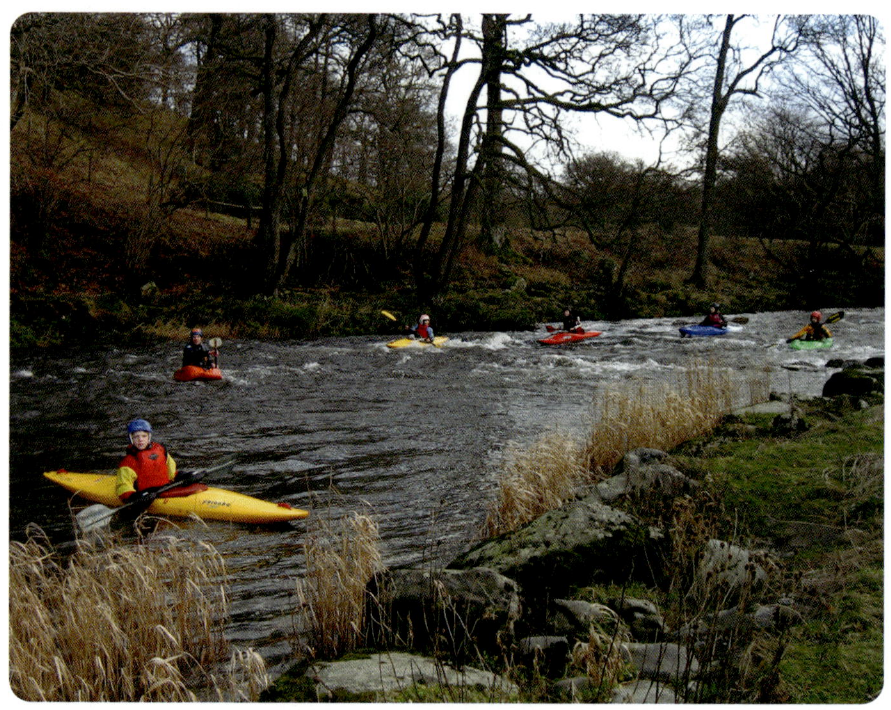

Canoeists on the River Greta

railway line and an impressive iron bridge. Pass through a kissing gate and up a short flight of steps to join the old railway track. Turn right, towards Keswick, crossing the first of four bridges dating from the 1860s which span the river.

Immediately after crossing the first bridge, a short diversion from the main track leads you to a hidden bench besides the river – a perfect spot for a picnic break.

5. From the picnic spot, retrace your steps to rejoin the old railway track. Turn right. The return leg is flat and easy to walk. It is part of the coast-to-coast cycle way which, due to its easy gradient, is very popular with local cyclists.

6. Cross over two more bridges. You may see trout and salmon gliding in the current under these bridges. On your right, after the third bridge, is Low Briery, now the location of a static caravan park, but previously the site of several mills that used the river to power their activities. Here the river has been harnessed for industrial purposes for six centuries. Bobbins used by the cotton and woollen industry were made at a bobbin mill which stood here until 1961, including those used to hold the thread for making the coronation gown worn by Queen Elizabeth II.

7. Continue following the track to yet another exciting part of the walk: the boardwalk section. The old railway line originally went through a tunnel at this point. On your left, just before the start of the boardwalk, you will see the outline of the top of an old tunnel which was blocked up many years ago. Your route continues by following the boardwalk, built over the steep ground that falls away towards the river. There are good views of the weir below from this elevated position.

8. The impressive Greta Bridge now comes into view again. A small monument, under the bridge, explains that the bridge was awarded the title of Best Concrete Engineering Structure of the Century.

On a clear day, you can see the area's finest peaks ahead of you. The knuckle-shaped summit of Causey Pike is easy to recognize and, as you get closer to Keswick, Cat Bells appears in the distance to your left and Skiddaw to your right.

9. The path descends towards Keswick, passing houses. Cross the final railway bridge of your walk. To your right are alpine-chalet style buildings, which are part of a time-share complex. You soon reach your final destination: the old Keswick railway station, complete with its defunct platform and ornate veranda. It is now part of the Keswick Hotel, but it is easy to think of it in its glory days when steam trains used to stop here.

10. Just past the old railway station is Keswick Pool and Fitness Centre, where you started your walk.

NEARBY ATTRACTION

Keswick is a popular tourist town with a wide variety of pubs, cafés, restaurants and other attractions. More information can be obtained from Keswick Tourist Information Centre, Moot Hall, Keswick, Cumbria, CA12 5JR, telephone: 017687 72645.

LOWESWATER

This walk leads you past old farmsteads and up onto the fellside to discover a beautiful, secluded tarn with tiny islands, on which heath spotted orchids grow in the summer months. The walk continues to a high point with wonderful views across Loweswater. You then go down the fellside and continue onto the lake shore, passing through attractive woodland.

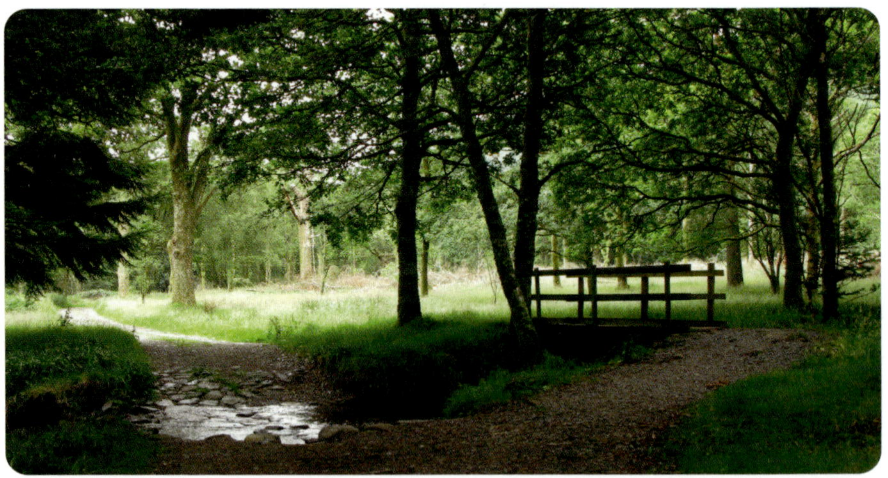

The route through Holme Wood

- **HOW TO GET THERE:** From Cockermouth follow the B5289 towards Buttermere, and then follow the road signed for Loweswater. As you reach the village, take the third turning on the left. This leads you down a narrow lane to Maggie's Bridge.
- **PARKING:** The car park at Maggie's Bridge where there is space for about eight cars (free of charge at the time of writing).
- **LENGTH OF WALK:** 5.3 miles/8.6 kilometres. **MAP:** OS Explorer OL4 and 303 (GR NY 134210).
- **TERRAIN:** A long section of gradual ascent followed by a descent to a level path along the lake-side section. A potentially toxic blue-green alga grows in the lake so do keep dogs and children out of the water.

Loweswater is off the beaten track and is one of the least visited of the Lake District's lakes. As a result, the valley still retains its old charm and is the perfect place to escape the crowds. The lake's name is derived from Old Scandinavian *lauf saer* 'leafy lake'. The lake is relatively small: just over a mile long and a third of a mile wide. The maximum depth of the lake is 59 feet, with an average depth of 27 feet.

Loweswater is a scattered collection of farmsteads, which are dotted around the lake. The centre of the village lies to the east of the lake. Here, the 16th-century Kirkstile Inn brews its own beers, provides good food and offers bed and breakfast accommodation. St Bartholomew's church stands opposite the pub. The church dates from 1884 and replaced a simple chapel which previously occupied the spot. Records from St Bees Priory indicate that there has been a place of worship in Loweswater from at least 1125. In the past, monks from the priory would conduct local services, and bodies would be taken away for burial along the corpse road through Holme Wood.

The annual Loweswater Show is a traditional agricultural event with an emphasis on livestock. It has run for over 130 years, taking place in September each year. The show also features fell races, Cumberland and Westmorland wrestling, sheep dog trials and hound trailing. Other attractions include a local craft fair and a variety of trade stands.

THE WALK

1. From the car park, ignore the track through the kissing gate which leads directly to the lake. Instead, walk a few metres back up the road that you travelled down to reach the car park, and then turn right along a track that passes over a small stone bridge known as Maggie's Bridge.

2. Continue along this track, which leads you up towards High Nook Farm. Your route initially sweeps to the left, through open fields, which are filled with colourful wild flowers in summer. Ahead of you is a small valley flanked by Gavel Fell, Blake Fell and Carling Knott. Pass a gate with *yat stoups*, gateposts that have several holes in them. Poles were slotted through the holes to form a barrier. The lowest pole could be removed to allow sheep to pass through.

3. Continue up the track. Ignore the turning on your right signed 'Watergate and Loweswater'. Cross the stream and then ascend slightly steeper terrain. Pass through High Nook Farm, an atmospheric farmstead which dates from the 16th century. Carry on through a wooden gate and

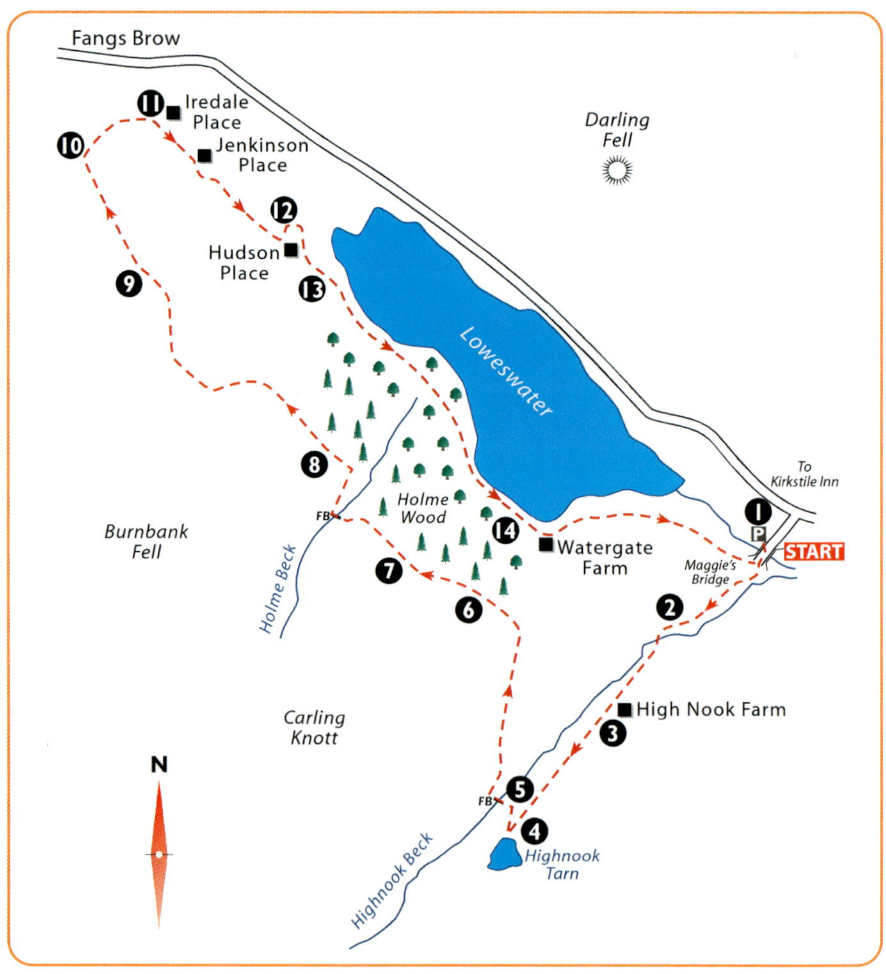

follow the path up the hillside. Highnook Beck flows down the valley on your right. When you reach the top of a steepish section, pass through another gate.

4. The path now becomes a grassy trod. Stick to the most obvious path, which runs parallel to the beck, and ignore the faint track which climbs the hillside on your left. The path is indistinct at this point and sometimes boggy. Continue walking roughly parallel to the stream – the path going through gaps in the bracken. After a few minutes you will reach Highnook Tarn on your left-hand side. This is a lovely setting: a picturesque mountain lake with a couple of tiny islands, where heath spotted orchids grow in summer.

5. You now need to cross to the other side of High Nook Beck: retrace your steps for a minute or so, and then descend towards the beck on a faint track. Cross the beck, using the small wooden bridge. Turn right and climb the path up the hillside. As you ascend you will now see Loweswater.

6. Continue climbing. A grassy terrace skirts the top of Holme Wood, which is filled with Scots pines. Just when you think you have reached the highest point of your walk there is a sting in the tail: another short steepish section. You might spot bilberries, which fruit in autumn, growing on the side of the path just before the next gate.

7. The gate marks the highpoint of your route, and you now start to descend. On a clear day, the Solway coast is visible in the distance ahead of you. Continue down the main track, ignoring the footpath which leads through the wood. Your route descends left towards Holme Beck. Cross the sturdy wooden sleeper bridge over Holme Beck and carry on.

8. You will reach a dilapidated wooden bench which stands in a commanding position overlooking the lake.

From here you are treated to a bird's-eye view of the lake and the surrounding valley. Crummock Water is also visible. The buoy which you can see in the middle of Loweswater analyses water samples as part of a research project which aims to reduce the incidence of the potentially toxic blue-green alga that grows in the lake.

9. Follow the path as it undulates across the fell side. Reach another gate, and then follow the track as it descends through rugged terrain, with a drystone wall on your right-hand side. In the near distance you may see the road known as Fangs Brow.

10. Some 200 metres before the road, take the footpath on your right. Follow the path indicated on the wooden fingerpost: 'public bridleway Loweswater via Hudson Place approximately 1 mile'. Your path descends through fields, following a drystone wall on the right. Continue through a metal gate and onto a rough track. You will see

Iredale Place, an old farmstead, through the trees on your left. Turn right; go up a slight incline and through a wooden gate, continuing in the direction of Loweswater. Follow the tarmac road, edged with trees.

11. At Jenkinson Place (an old farmstead), turn right and go up a rough track; go through a gate and onto a track which then cuts through fields. Through the field follow the faint path which goes through a gap in the stone wall ahead. Now, follow a row of old hawthorns and the remains of an old drystone wall. You soon reach another gate and stile in a shady spot beside two small streams.

12. Go into the next field and head towards Hudson Place. Turn left, through a wooden gate and stile, immediately before reaching this old farmstead. A weathered stone footpath sign and a bridleway badge on the gatepost point the way. Gradually descend through a field and head towards a wooden gate. You will reach a tarmac road with a fingerpost in front of you. Turn right here and follow the road as it passes in front of Hudson Place. Continue on this road until you reach two gates.

13. When you reach the gates, take the left-hand gate displaying the footpath sign. Descend along a rough track which narrows as you get closer to the lake. Go through a wooden gate and on to the side of the lake. Keep on. Your route now follows the obvious track through Holme Wood.

En route, you will pass a stone building beside the lake, known as Holme Wood Bothy. This is a converted fish hatchery, owned by the National Trust, which can be booked for overnight stays.

14. The track eventually leaves the wood, and Watergate Farm comes into view. The wide grassy area in front of the farm is popular with picnickers. Continue along the track to the car park where you started your walk.

NEARBY ATTRACTIONS
The town of **Cockermouth** and the **Whinlatter Visitor Centre**, at the top of Whinlatter Pass (B5292), are both within easy reach. Cockermouth Tourist Information can be contacted at the Town Hall, Market Street, Cockermouth, CA13 9NP, telephone: 01900 822 634. **Kirkstile Inn**, Loweswater, telephone: 01900 85219.

THIRLMERE

After a short ascent of the hillside overlooking Thirlmere, the route traverses the landscape, passing three attractive waterfalls before descending towards the lake. The path then follows the shoreline through pleasant woodland, which includes atmospheric Greathow Wood, where red deer are known to raise their young.

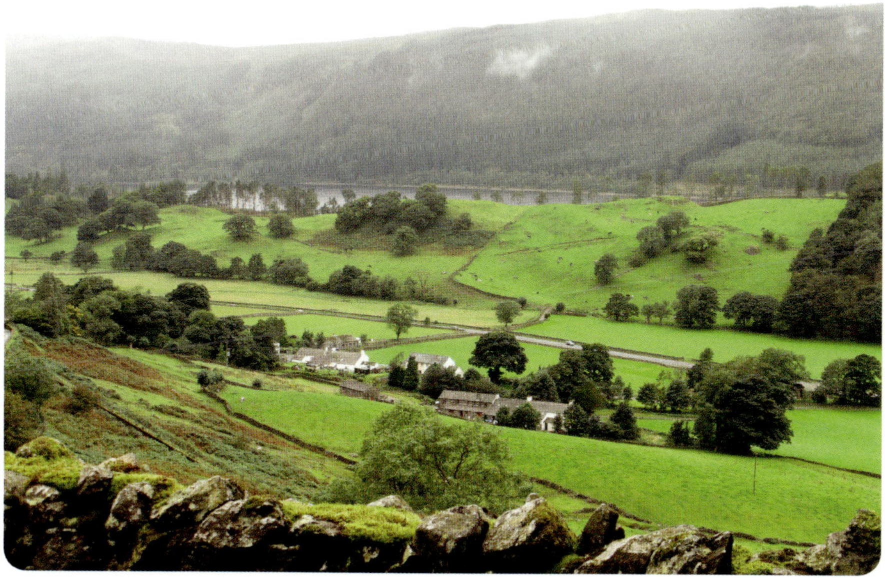

The view towards Thirlmere

- **HOW TO GET THERE:** From Keswick or Grasmere follow the A591. A small pull-in is located on the Keswick side of the junction for the B5322.
- **PARKING:** The roadside pull-in which has space for about six cars.
- **LENGTH OF WALK:** 4.3 miles/7.0 kilometres. **MAP:** OS Explorer OL5 (GR NY 318189).
- **TERRAIN:** Rough paths along the hillside, narrow in places and sometimes muddy; undulating woodland trails through the lake-shore section.

Thirlmere is a reservoir which supplies water to Manchester, 95 miles away. It has a capacity of 9,000 million gallons and can supply 50 million gallons of water per day. The dam's foundation stone was laid in 1890, and the structure was built from stone quarried in Longridge, Lancashire, and delivered by train to a specially constructed railway siding at Windermere station. The dam raised the water level by 50 feet. The opening ceremony took place on 12th October 1894 and the commemorative stone can be seen by the side of the road on the dam head. The project cost £1.5 million.

The flooding of the valley swallowed up Leathes Water, which lay in the bottom of the valley. Leathes Water was named after the ancient Leathes family at Dale Head, who once owned the surrounding land. The old lake was split into two parts by a narrow peninsula. A shallow, fast-flowing river joined the two parts, and shepherds used an oak plank bridge with a wooden handrail to cross the river and reach the other side of the valley. Leathes Water was also known as Wythburn Water, after the small hamlet located at the southern end of the lake.

The flooding of the valley ran into opposition from the Thirlmere Defence Association. John Ruskin, the Victorian poet, artist and conservationist stated that 'Manchester should be put to the bottom of Thirlmere'.

THE WALK

1. Leave the car parking area by the exit which leads onto the B5322. Walk up the B5322 for approximately 50 metres and then turn right, up Stanah Lane, following the fingerpost for 'bridleway Glenridding via Sticks Pass'. Pass beside Thirlmere Recreation Hall. Ascend the lane until you reach the end of a large stone barn on your left (where the lane bends to the left). You will see a five-step stile in front of you.

2. Climb the stile, signed 'Sticks Pass', over the wall. The path then climbs up a steepish section of field. The route bears right and crosses a stile beside a wooden gate near a rocky outcrop. Go up to the rough path that climbs the hillside. Pass through a wooden gate to reach a series of waterfalls at Sty Beck.

3. The path now bears right, in front of the falls, and then ascends the hillside. A fingerpost indicates 'public footpath Swirls car park'. Your route bends to the right and follows a stone wall. Initially, the high wall blocks your view across the valley, but it then becomes lower, allowing

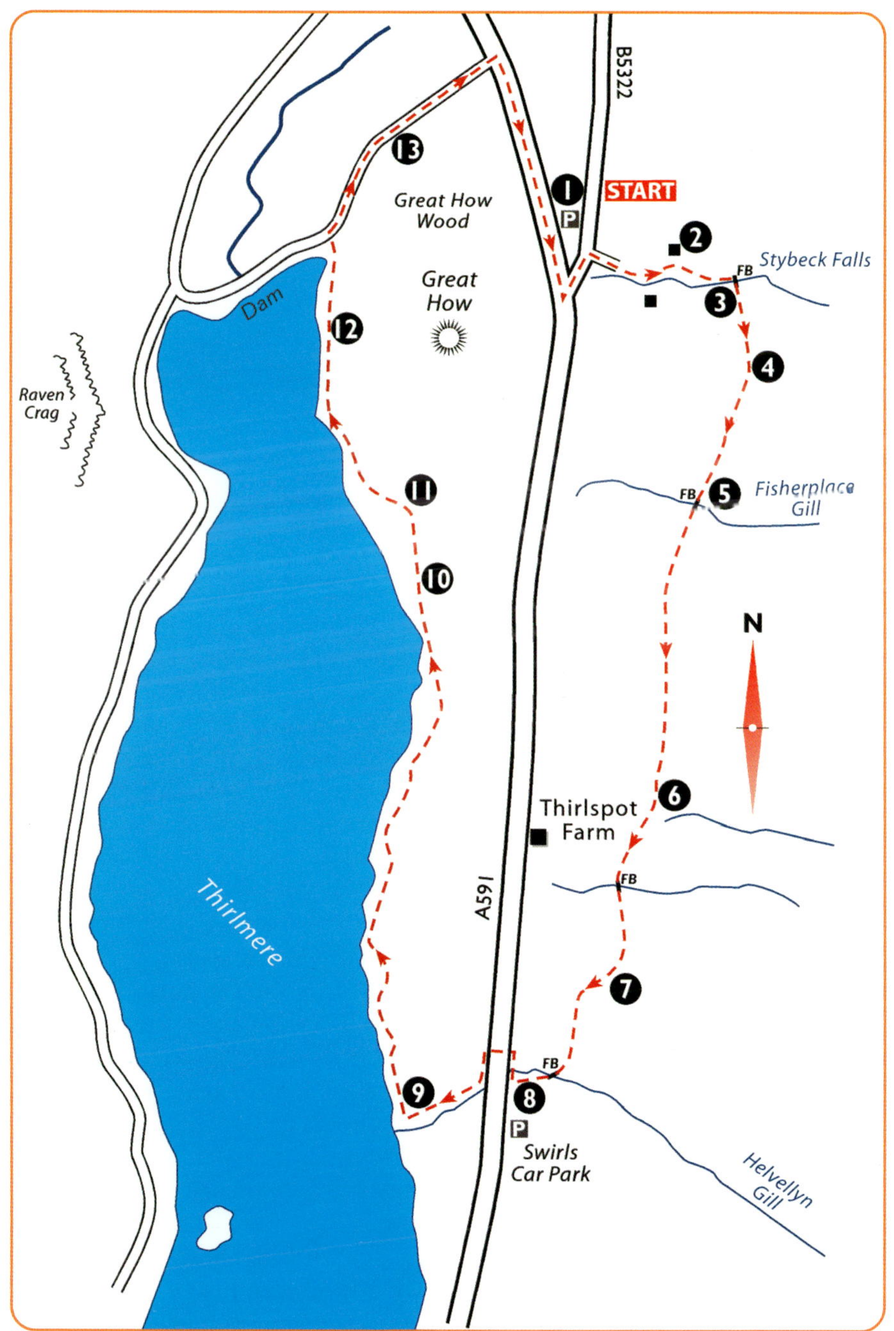

B5322
START
P
1
2
Stybeck Falls
FB
3
4
Great How Wood
Great How
Dam
12
13
Raven Crag
FB
5
Fisherplace Gill
11
10
N
Thirlmere
6
Thirlspot Farm
FB
A591
7
FB
8
9
FB
P
Swirls Car Park
Helvellyn Gill

you to see the wooded slopes of Great How. Proceed along the narrow, sometimes muddy, path.

4. When you reach a low wooden guidepost, keep straight on. Do not follow the narrow paths that descend the hillside on your right.

5. You will reach another attractive waterfall beside a sturdy wooden bridge at Fisherplace Gill. Cross the bridge and continue to follow the path.

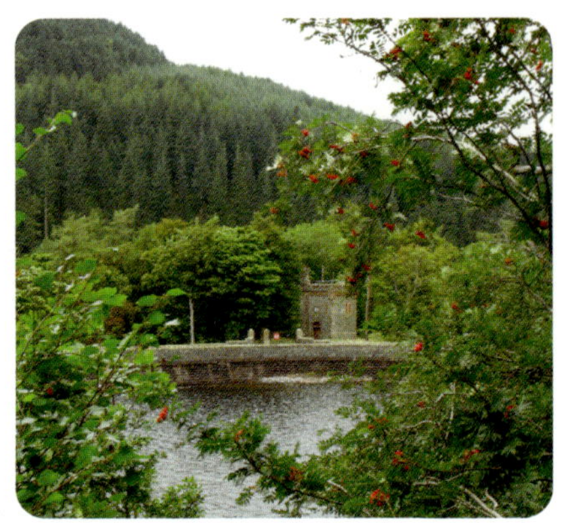

The dam wall can be seen from the path

There are good views across Thirlmere from this section of your walk. On a fine day, Skiddaw can also be seen in the distance, on the right.

6. You will reach a small beck with an etched slate sign just before it. Keep straight ahead, following the fingerpost 'public footpath Swirls car park and Helvellyn', and ignoring the path that goes right. Make your way along a rocky path, which climbs initially, before starting to descend. Thirlspot Farm is visible below you. The path now descends more sharply until you reach a small wooden footbridge across another beck with waterfalls. Continue over a rocky section towards Swirls car park, which you may see ahead of you, in the middle distance.

7. The path climbs again and then descends. You will arrive at the corner of a stone wall with a fingerpost in front of you. Descend to the right here, dropping down through the field, towards the car park. Go across a small wooden bridge and then through a kissing gate. Pass through another gate and then go over another wooden bridge, which crosses Helvellyn Gill. Turn right into the car park area. Toilets are available here.

8. From the car park proceed towards the main road (A591), and then turn right. Walk along the side of the road for a short distance until you reach another parking area on the opposite side of the road. Go through the car park in the direction of the lake, descending some steps. Ignore the gate which is immediately in front of you; instead turn left and pass through a kissing gate beside the wooden gate. Follow the sign for 'permissive lakeshore path – The Dam, The How, Legburthwaite'. Descend through the field. The path joins a wooden fence beside a powerful section of beck, with cascades.

9. Descend further; go through a kissing gate and follow the side of the beck. You will see the lake shore through the trees in front of you. The path bears right and carries on through mixed woodland. Pass through a small clearing and then re-enter the woods. Keep left at a white waymarker and stick to the main path.

10. The path now leaves the lake shore and climbs up along a broader track through a forest clearing. Pass through a kissing gate beside a wooden gate. Your route now climbs slightly, passing wiry silver birch trees.

11. You will reach a crossroads in the path, in front of the wooded hill known as Great How. Look for the four-way fingerpost. Turn left and follow the sign to the dam. Descend towards the lake shore along the path. The track soon bears right, following the lake shore into a dense oak wood. Make your way through the wood, keeping an eye out for red deer. You are advised to keep dogs on leads.

12. You will start to see the dam wall ahead of you, and Raven Crag can be seen rising majestically on the other side of the lake. Descend a short rocky section with a handrail beside it. Take care; it can be a bit tricky. Cross over three sections of boarding that span wet ground and continue. You will reach a kissing gate and then steps that go down to the road and a fingerpost. When you reach the road go right.

13. Follow the road, passing a slate-covered building on your left and then Bridge End Farm, with its caravan and camp site. You will soon reach the main road, the A591. Turn right along the A591 and walk along the grass verge. After several minutes you will reach your starting point on the opposite side of the road.

NEARBY ATTRACTIONS

Keswick is a popular tourist town with a wide variety of pubs, cafés, restaurants and other attractions. More information can be obtained from Keswick Tourist Information Centre, Moot Hall, Keswick, Cumbria, CA12 5JR, telephone: 01768 772645.

ENNERDALE WATER AND RIVER LIZA

This route follows the lakeside, with striking views across Ennerdale Water, and then heads into a less frequented area, higher up the valley. You pass near the towering cliffs of Pillar Rock, and then continue alongside the beautiful River Liza, through the site of an Iron Age settlement and past a Bronze Age cairn field, before returning along the lake shore.

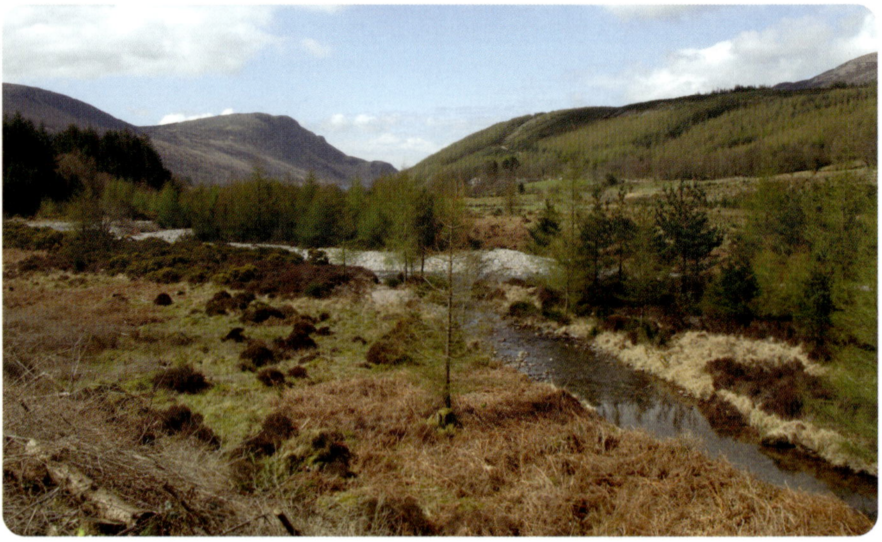

The beautiful River Liza

- **HOW TO GET THERE:** From the A5086 follow the signs for Ennerdale Bridge. In Ennerdale Bridge follow signs for Croasdale and The Lake. Continue past the turning for Broadmoor to a car park.
- **PARKING:** Bowness Knott free car park next to Ennerdale Water.
- **LENGTH OF WALK:** 8.1 miles/12.9 kilometres. **MAP:** OS Explorer OL4 and 303 (GR NY 109153).
- **TERRAIN:** Mostly flat, with some gentle climbs. The route mainly follows obvious tracks. Extra care should be taken on the short section of path besides the rapids just after the bridge over the River Liza.

Getting to Ennerdale isn't easy, but your efforts will be rewarded once you arrive. It is the most westerly of the Lake District lakes and is reached by travelling along winding country lanes. Very few people live in the valley and the number of visitors is low, allowing you to find peace and solitude. The scenery is superb and has a wild, rugged feel.

The valley holds the most impressive collection of Bronze Age (2000 BC to 800 BC) and domestic medieval and post-medieval (AD 410 to 1600) archaeology in the Lake District. Archaeologists, surveying the valley between 1995 and 2003, identified a total 552 individual monuments during their research. These included a cairn field, located at the eastern end of the lake, thought to be of Bronze Age origin; an Iron Age settlement on the south bank of the River Liza; and several bloomeries – furnaces fuelled with charcoal to produce wrought iron.

Roe deer can be spotted near the lake in the early morning, and the rarer red deer is slowly moving into the area too. Badgers, foxes and red squirrels live in the woodland that surrounds the lake. Peregrine falcons nest on the nearby crags, and salmon occasionally climb the fish ladder into the lake on their journey to spawn. A rare and genetically distinct species of arctic charr lives in the lake, and can sometimes be seen flickering along the gravel beds of streams that feed the lake, which they enter at night to spawn.

THE WALK

1. From Bowness Knott car park, join the forest track and turn left along it. The road descends towards Ennerdale Lake. The lake will be on your right.

On the opposite side of the lake, you will see the rocky outcrop of Anglers Crag. Ahead of you, in the distance, are the impressive mountains of Pillar, Scoat Fell and Haycock. The views of the lake now begin to open out and on a clear day you may even see Great Gable at the head of the valley.

2. Carry on along the track. Pass the fingerpost for the Smithy Beck Trail on your left.

As you cross Smithy Beck itself, look to your right for slight undulations in the ground, circular in shape. This is the site of a medieval bloomery.

When you reach the end of the lake, you will see the River Liza, which

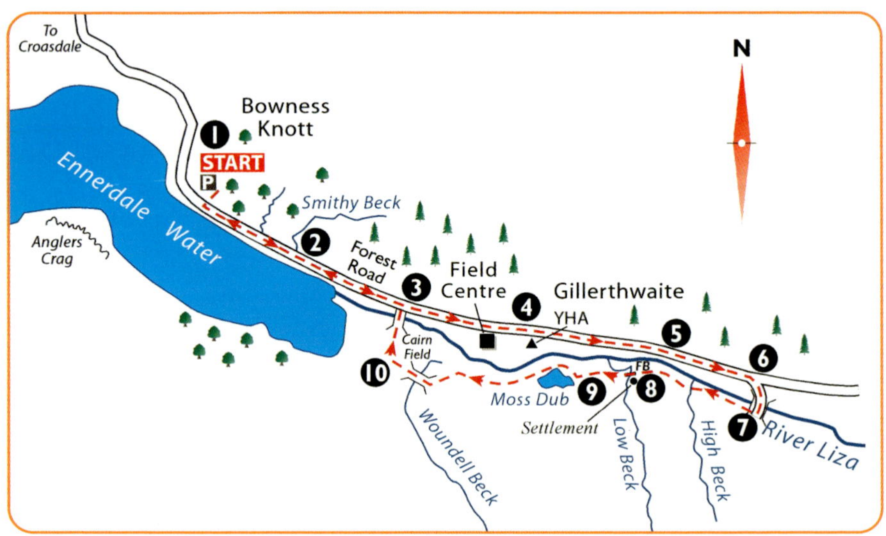

has tumbled down the valley, joining the lake. Carry on. A riverside path runs for a short distance upstream and is a pleasant alternative to the track which runs alongside.

3. A low concrete bridge which crosses the river soon comes into view on your right. Ignore this turning; your route carries on up the valley. (You will eventually cross this bridge on the return leg of your walk.) Your route now climbs gently, passing areas of mixed woodland to your left and overlooking open fields on your right. As you make progress, you will see the river bending away from you to your right. At this point, the river is a broad, rocky flash along the valley bottom.

4. As you approach Low Gillerthwaite Field Centre, you will pass a stile that has climbing rope as tread for its steps. Next, you pass the Youth Hostel, which nestles in a stand of Scots pines. This area was once the site of a medieval community.

5. A fork in the track now appears. Ignore the track on the left and keep straight on.

You should see the impressive peaks of Pillar, Scoat Fell and Haycock rising above the valley on your right, unless the valley is covered with low cloud.

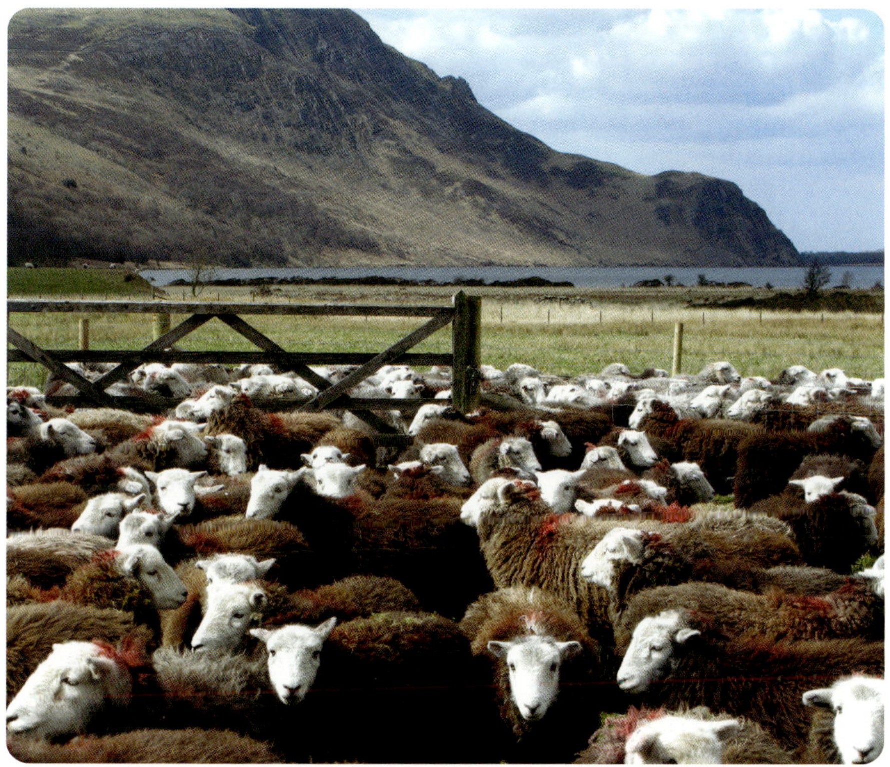

Herdwick sheep are a common sight on the Lakeland fells

Continue through a gate at Gillerthwaite. Once again, the river starts to converge with your track.

6. Continue along the main track, ignoring the minor tracks on your left. When you reach a major fork in the track, take the right fork, signed 'Pillar'. This leads to a bridge over the River Liza, which crashes down the valley in a series of powerful falls and deep pools here. This is a beautiful setting. Above you are the spectacular cliffs of Pillar Rock, and there are views back towards the lake and Anglers Crag.

7. Turn right immediately after crossing the bridge to follow the narrow path along the edge of the river. Take care along this riverside section. After a few metres you will come to some boulders and a concrete block. This is a perfect picnic stop, with excellent views of the pools and falls.

8. Follow the path downstream. The river here is spectacular. The path is a little obscure in places, and occasionally boggy after heavy rainfall. Cross the footbridge which spans High Beck. The path bends slightly right, following the river and passing a ruin on your left. The path now veers left, away from the river. Pass through a new gate and cross two more footbridges at Low Beck.

You will now see crescent-shaped raised banking close to the river. This is the location of an Iron Age settlement.

Carry on. As your path climbs, your elevated position offers good views of the river and across the valley. Proceed along the undulating, occasionally muddy, path which goes through the woods.

9. Turn right when you meet another path and make a short descent towards a shallow lake called Moss Dubb. Continue through the atmospheric pine woods, and then turn right when you meet a forest track. Pass through a gate with a cattle grid, and then cross a low concrete bridge over Woundell Beck. Continue through an area of tall Scots pines.

10. When you reach a T-junction in the track, turn right and pass through another gate with a cattle grid. Follow this short, straight section of forest track.

Look for patches of boulders buried in the field on your right. These are believed to be Bronze Age cairns.

Cross the river over the low concrete bridge that you passed at the start of your walk. Turn left and retrace your steps along the track, back to Bowness Knott car park.

NEARBY ATTRACTIONS

The towns of **Cockermouth** and **Whitehaven** are located nearby. Cockermouth Tourist Information Centre can be contacted at the Town Hall, Market Street, Cockermouth, CA13 9NP, telephone: 01900 822 634. Whitehaven Tourist Information Centre is based at Market Hall, Whitehaven, CA28 7JG, telephone: 01946 852 939. The **Shepherds Arms**, Ennerdale Bridge, telephone: 01946 861 249.

BUTTERMERE

You set off from the village of Buttermere, an attractive, unspoilt, less busy part of the Lake District. Your route then follows the lakeshore, taking you through pleasant woodland and past pebbly bays. High mountains flank the lake and waterfalls shimmer down the fellside.

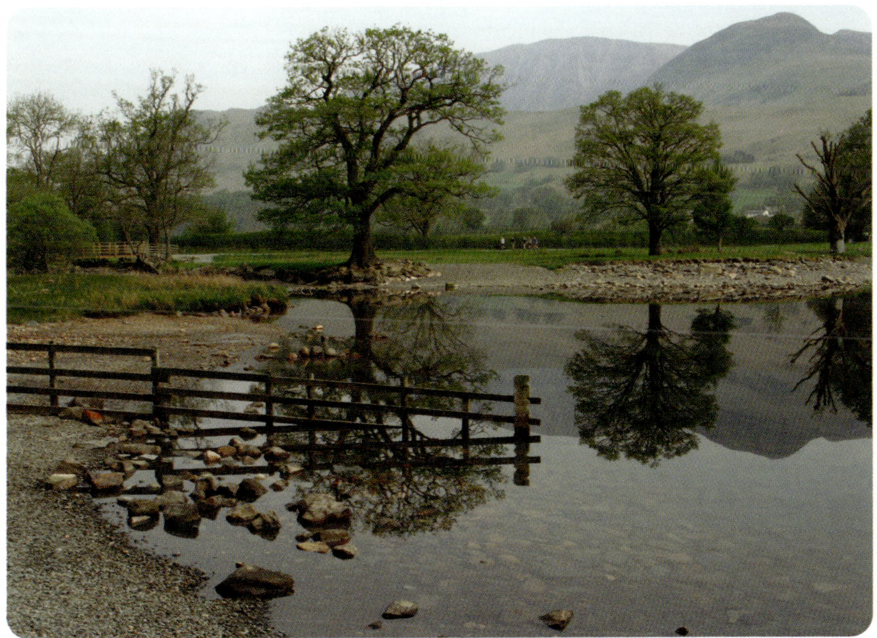

Buttermere Lake is owned by the National Trust

- **HOW TO GET THERE:** From Cockermouth or Keswick follow the B5289 into the village until you reach the Bridge Hotel. Turn down the road at the side of the hotel and head towards the Fish Hotel.
- **PARKING:** The National Trust pay-and-display car park near the hotel.
- **LENGTH OF WALK:** 4.5 miles/7.2 kilometres. **MAP:** OS Explorer OL4 (GR NY 173169).
- **TERRAIN:** The walk is mainly flat and uses obvious paths.

41

Buttermere is a small village situated between the lakes of Buttermere and Crummock Water. The name Buttermere means 'lake by dairy pastures' from Old English *'butere mere'*. Buttermere Lake is owned by The National Trust. It is 1.2 miles long and 0.3 mile wide and has a maximum depth of 94 feet. The village has two pubs, a tea shop, several holiday cottages, a campsite and a youth hostel.

The small parish church of St James stands overlooking the village. Inside, a stone tablet set into a windowsill is a memorial to Alfred Wainwright, the famous fell walker, illustrator and author of walking guidebooks. The window looks out towards his favourite mountain, Haystacks, where his ashes were scattered in 1991.

The Fish Hotel was the scene of a scandal in 1802. Mary, the innkeeper's pretty teenage daughter, had become known as the 'Beauty of Buttermere' after being mentioned in a guide book that was written some years earlier. She attracted visitors who had read about her charms. In 1802, a man passing himself off as the Honourable Alexander Augustus Hope, brother of the Earl of Hopetoun, and the Member of Parliament for Linlithgow, stayed at the inn. He courted Mary and they were married at Lorton church on 2nd October, 1802. It was soon discovered that her husband was an impostor, a notorious swindler, felon and bigamist whose real name was John Hatfield. He took flight, and notices were printed in national publications offering a £50 reward for his capture. He was eventually apprehended by Bow Street officers 16 miles from Swansea and brought to trial at the Cumberland Assizes on 15th August, 1803. Hatfield was tried on charges that included impersonating a Member of Parliament and forgery. He was found guilty and was later hanged in Carlisle.

THE WALK

1. From the Fish Hotel, go past the Bridge Hotel and then take the road which bears right and climbs uphill. After 75 metres, turn right at Syke House Farm; a fingerpost directs you to the lake-shore path and bridleway. You will pass a shop well known for its excellent ice cream. Keep straight ahead; go through the farmyard, passing a couple of old barns; and pass through a gate.

2. Carry on along the track, passing a cattle trough and a gate. A National Trust sign asks you to keep dogs on a lead. You will soon see Buttermere down to your right. Across the lake, on the fellside, you will see a waterfall tumbling down Sourmilk Gill. Continue on the track through fields.

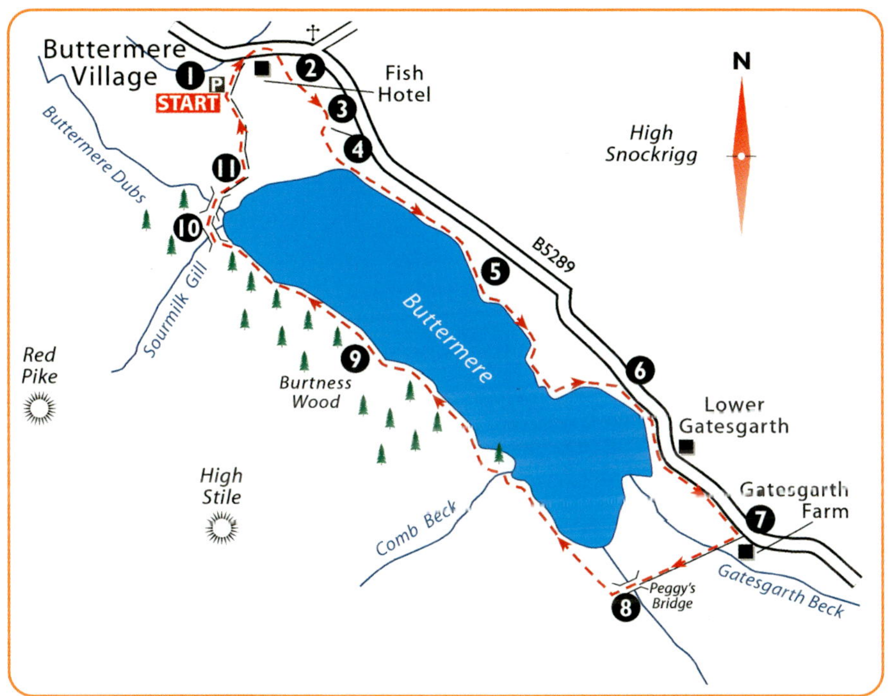

3. Just before you reach a large gate at the end of the second major field, turn right through a small gate which displays a small sign: 'shoreline path'. You will now descend towards the lake on a footpath between hedges.

4. You will soon reach a point overlooking a small pebbly bay.

This bay is closed from 1st April to 30th June to allow the common sandpiper to nest. It spends the winter overseas in Africa, South Asia and Australasia, and returns to the UK to bring up its young.

Follow the main path through mixed woodland as it runs approximately parallel to the lake shore.

5. Stick to the main path, ignoring any minor paths which join the main route round the lake. Your route takes you through an intriguing tunnel that cuts through the rock next to the lake, and then across a footbridge and into an area of Scots pines with good views of the head of the lake.

As you progress, you will see the frequently photographed Buttermere pines, which stand along the lake shore.

6. Continue on the path until you reach the road. Turn right and follow the road for just over 600 metres.

On your way, you pass Lower Gatesgarth, formerly the home of Sir Claude Aurelius Elliott OBE, who was headmaster of Eton College between 1933 and 1949, and provost from 1949 to 1965.

7. The road now descends towards Gatesgarth Farm. When the road crosses Gatesgarthdale Beck, turn right to follow the fingerpost marked 'Public Bridleway, Buttermere and Ennerdale'. Go through the gate which displays a small sign for 'lakeside path', and then follow public bridleway and lakeside path signs. Your path follows Gatesgarthdale Beck for a short distance, and then becomes a broad, straight track, which leads you towards the opposite side of the valley. You will see Buttermere in the near distance, to your right.

8. Cross the wooden bridge known as Peggy's Bridge. Pass through a kissing gate and then turn right, towards the lake. Stick to the obvious path, which follows the lakeside.

9. Continue over the wooden footbridge and keep right, and then head into the shady pine trees of Burtness Wood. Keep on; your route follows the rocky lake shore, passing more pebbly bays.

10. Buttermere village soon comes into view in the middle distance ahead of you. Continue through the woods until you approach the end of the lake. Turn right through a gate and across a small footbridge which spans the beck that flows down Sourmilk Gill. Next, go over a more substantial bridge that crosses the river which flows out of the lake.

11. Continue along the short, straight track before turning left. Carry on until you reach the Fish Hotel.

NEARBY ATTRACTIONS
Honister Slate Mine is situated at the top of Honister Pass (B5289). It has a café, visitor centre, and runs mine tours. The **Fish Hotel** (telephone: 017687 70253), the **Bridge Hotel** (telephone: 017687 70252).

LANGSTRATH BECK FROM STONETHWAITE

This walk explores wild and remote Langstrath Valley. The route leads you beside rocky Stonethwaite and Langstrath becks, towards the head of this wide and rugged valley, which is reminiscent of a Scottish glen. The landscape is windswept and hauntingly beautiful. A sense of space and solitude prevails.

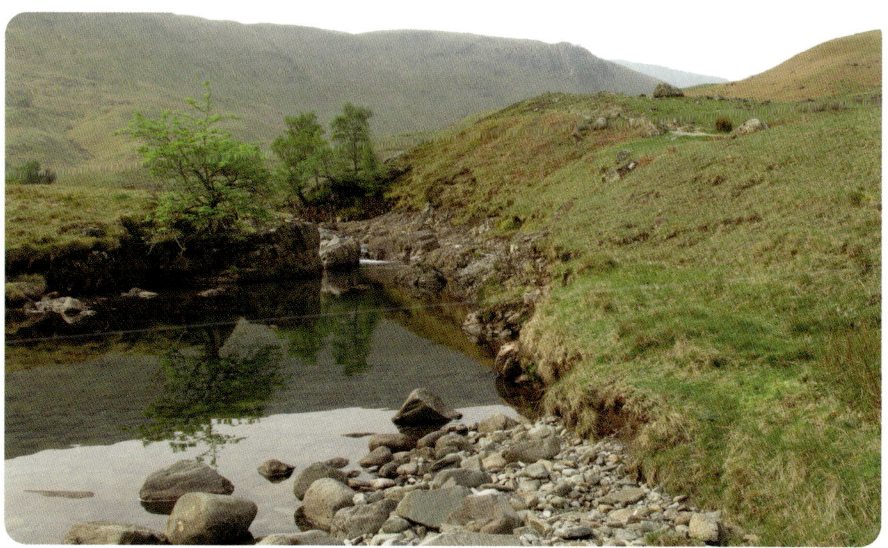

Langstrath Beck at Swan Dub

- **HOW TO GET THERE:** From Keswick follow the B5289 along the eastern shore of Derwentwater and down into Borrowdale. After you have passed through the hamlet of Rosthwaite, turn left, following signs for Stonethwaite and Langstrath Country Inn.
- **PARKING:** The roadside pull-in on the right just before Stonethwaite village where there is a limited number of parking spaces.
- **LENGTH OF WALK:** 6.5 miles/10.4 kilometres. **MAP:** OS Explorer OL4 (GR NY 260139).
- **TERRAIN:** The route follows rugged paths, with some wet sections.

Fountains Abbey had owned the Langstrath Valley since 1195 when, in 1209, the rest of Borrowdale was sold to Furness Abbey. Both abbeys laid claim to the rich pasture land surrounding Stonethwaite, and this developed into a major land dispute. In 1304 King Edward I intervened and confiscated the land. Later, the monks from Fountains Abbey outsmarted their Cumbrian rivals by purchasing the land from the Crown for 40 shillings, and managed the land from their abbey near Ripon.

The village of Stonethwaite was built for the local miners and farm workers. The village pub, the Langstrath Country Inn, was originally a cottage that was built around 1590 and called Dove Cottage. The remains of the old cottage are visible in the restaurant in its original doorways and low oak lintels.

An area known as Ore Gap lies at the head of Langstrath Valley. The ground is stained red by haematite. In medieval times iron ore was mined here by the monks of Fountains Abbey and then transported the length of the valley to an iron smelter on Smithymire Island, at the confluence of Greenup Gill and Langstrath Beck. Your outward journey takes you close to the site of the former smelter. A visible remnant from the past is the ruined building near the bridge over Langstrath Beck, which you pass on your return leg. It was once an inn known as 'Auld Jwonny Hoose', which was run by Johnny around the beginning of the 19th century. It is marked as 'Johnny House' on OS maps.

THE WALK

1. From the parking space, walk along the road towards the village until you see a red telephone box and a wooden fingerpost. Go left here, following the footpath sign to Greenup Edge and Grasmere. Continue along the rough track between two stone walls, passing an information board about Herdwick sheep. You will soon reach a bridge that spans Stonethwaite Beck.

2. Cross the bridge and go through a gate. You will reach another fingerpost. Turn right here and join the public bridleway to Grasmere via Greenup Edge. Continue along the rocky track and go through a gate. You will pass a well constructed sheep fold on your left.

3. Pass through a gate and continue along the rough track, which bends to the left and then crosses a small sleeper bridge. You will pass beside a small ruin. The track then narrows and descends slightly. The rapids

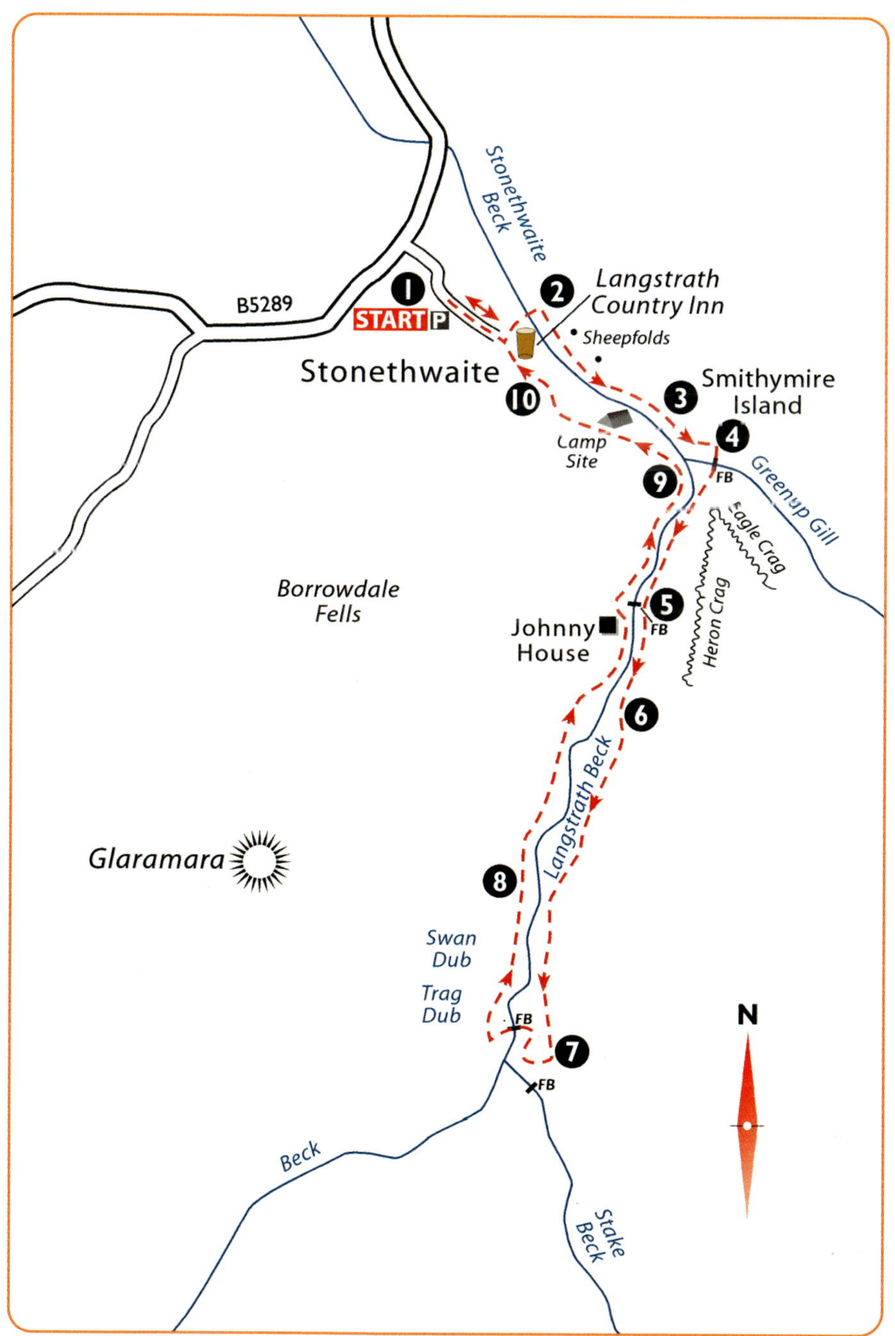

Stonethwaite Beck
B5289
START P
1
2 Langstrath Country Inn
Sheepfolds
Stonethwaite
10
3 Smithymire Island
4
Camp Site
9
FB
Greenup Gill
Eagle Crag
Heron Crag
Borrowdale Fells
5 FB
Johnny House
6
Langstrath Beck
Glaramara
8
Swan Dub
Trag Dub
FB
7
FB
N
Beck
Stake Beck

soon come into view on your right. Proceed along the path, passing another sheepfold.

4.   You will see that the valley splits ahead of you and you will reach the confluence of two becks which run down the valleys of Greenup and Langstrath. The area at the confluence of the two becks is Smithymire Island. Your route bears right and follows Langstrath Valley. Look out for the path which goes right and crosses the beck at a wooden footbridge. Follow this path, ignoring the one that carries on into Greenup Valley. A brass plaque on the bridge informs you that the bridge was re-erected in memory of Gordon Hallworth, a member of Manchester University Mountaineering Club, who died of exhaustion in the valley in January 1939. A beautiful deep pool is located just over the bridge on your right.

5.   Press on up the valley, following the main path.

Across to your right is the river, with a series of cascades and pools, an enchanting spot which tempts you to stay all day.

You will soon reach a footbridge over Langstrath Beck. Ignore this turning and keep going straight on. To your left are good views of the gnarled face of Heron Crag. On your right, shallow Langstrath Beck flows over a rocky bed.

6.   You will see a huge perched stone block, known as Blea Rock, ahead of you. A rising rocky path skirts the knoll on which it sits. Carry on past the boulder and then climb a stile over a stone wall near the river. Ignore the path through the gate. There are now extensive views up the valley. On the opposite side of the valley is Cam Crag. Carry on past a series of six cairns.

7.   Carry on up the valley. Turn right immediately before the footbridge that crosses Stake Beck and follow the beck downstream until it reaches Langstrath Beck. Head downstream for a short distance and then cross the footbridge which spans the small, impressive gorge. Once over, turn right and now descend the valley on the other side of Langstrath Beck. Pass Tray Dub and Swan Dub. Dub indicates a pool or deep water in a beck. The river bank below Swan Dub is a good place for a break and a picnic.

8. Continue down the rocky path, passing another series of cairns. You will reach a broad grassy area. Proceed towards a stone wall. A gate in the wall, located not far from the river, leads you onto another stony trail.

The old ruin on your left, just before the footbridge over Langstrath Beck, which you passed earlier, was once an inn known as 'Auld Jwonny Hoose'.

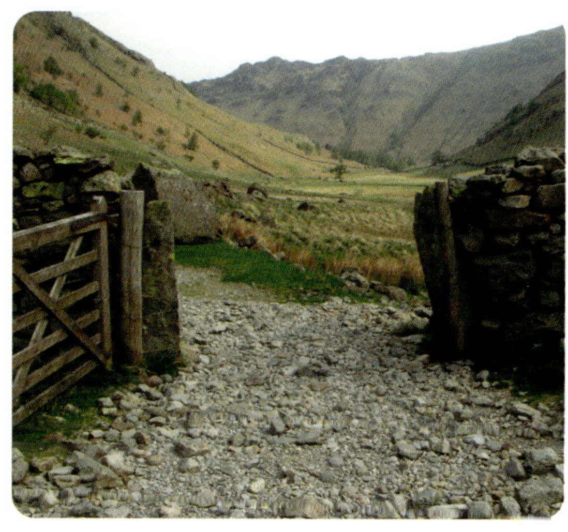
The path leading down the valley

Continue past a large boulder that is set into the stone wall. To your right are attractive pools and cascades shaded by overhanging trees.

9. Ignore a faint path on your right and continue down the main track alongside the stone wall. This avoids the campsite.

10. You will reach the Langstrath Country Inn, which serves good beers and food. A humorous plaque on the wall reminds you of prevailing weather conditions in the valley. Just past the pub is a tea shop that is open during summer months. Carry on until you reach the phone box, which you passed at the beginning of your walk. Bear left here to return to your starting point.

NEARBY ATTRACTIONS

The **Bowder Stone** is a delicately balanced 2,000-ton stone, which is 30 feet high, 50 feet wide and 90 feet in circumference. It is one of the Lake District's most famous attractions. It is located a short walk from a signed car park, just off the A590, south of the village of Grange. The **Langstrath Country Inn**, telephone: 01768 777239.

WET SLEDDALE RESERVOIR

Your route follows a circuit around Wet Sleddale dam. This walk gets you away from it all and leads you across a rugged landscape with big skies and a sense of space. Adders and red deer are sometimes seen in the area. En route, the track passes over a footbridge and past Wet Sleddal Hall.

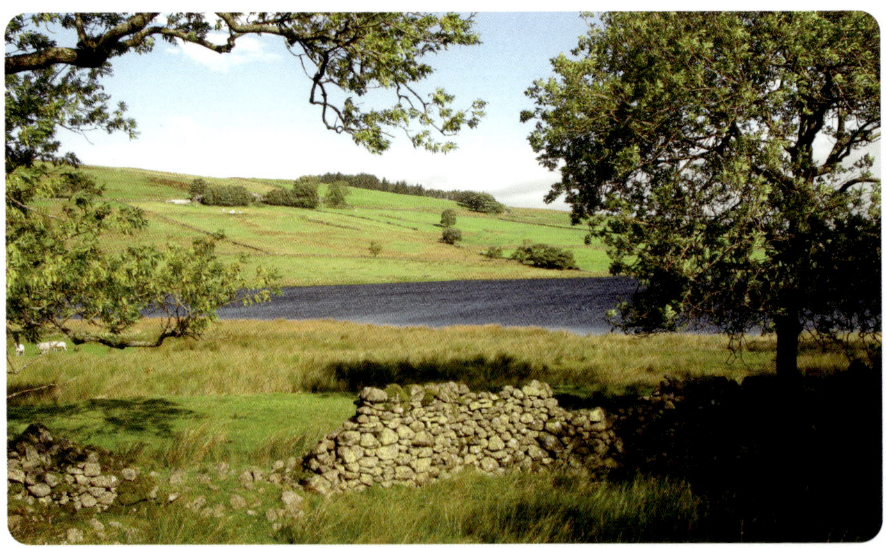

Wet Sleddale – pretty as a picture

- **HOW TO GET THERE:** From junction 39 of the M6, follow signs to Shap. Turn right along the A6, towards Shap. Take the next turning left, signed 'Wet Sleddale'. Follow the road, which bears left towards the corner of the dam wall.
- **PARKING:** The free car park near the dam wall.
- **LENGTH OF WALK:** 3.2 miles/5.2 kilometres. **MAP:** OS Explorer OL5 (GR NY 554114).
- **TERRAIN:** Mainly obvious paths, with some boggy sections after wet weather, and a couple of short uphill sections. Ground nesting birds and adders are present so please keep dogs on leads.

The hamlet of Sleddale was distinguished from the other Sleddale near Kendal by the addition of the epithet Wet. In days gone by, it was said that 'if any rain is stirring, the air scoops it surprisingly into the hollow of that dale'. The wet valley was the ideal choice for a reservoir, and construction started on a dam in the 1960s. It was completed in 1967 to supplement the nearby reservoir of Haweswater. The plain mass concrete dam at Wet Sleddale is 70 ft high and has a capacity of 500 million gallons.

Wet Sleddale was the location for the 1986 British film, *Withnail and I*. This was Richard E. Grant's first film role and launched him on a successful career. The film featured performances by Richard Griffiths as Withnail's Uncle Monty, Paul McGann as 'I' and Ralph Brown as Danny the drug dealer. The route crosses the bridge where Withnail and Marwood go 'fishing' in the film and passes the dilapidated Sleddale Hall, which was used as Monty's cottage, *Crow Crag*.

Adders are at large in the area and warning signs advise you to keep dogs on a short lead. The adder is Britain's only poisonous snake and can be recognized by the distinctive dark zigzag pattern which runs down the length of their spine. They are not aggressive animals and will only use their poison as a last means of defence, usually if handled or trodden on.

THE WALK

1. Leave the car park and walk up the track, passing the end of the dam wall. Continue along the track and then go through a metal gate. You will soon reach a fork in the path; keep straight on, ignoring the path which bears left towards a barn. At this point there are good views across the reservoir and towards the low fells at the other side of the valley.

2. On your right pass a small wooded area enclosed by a fence. You will approach a dilapidated barn on your right, partly hidden in the trees. A small marker post directs you along the footpath that forks left here. However, this section is very boggy; so keep to the other path, which goes straight on, passing near the old building. Then cross the modern wooden footbridge and, immediately after, turn left and pass between the end of a stone wall and the stream. This will get you back on course.

3. Your route continues ahead, ascending as you go. To your right is a stone wall. Pass a notice reminding you to keep dogs on a lead and to stick to the paths. The path goes through a gap in the wall and continues

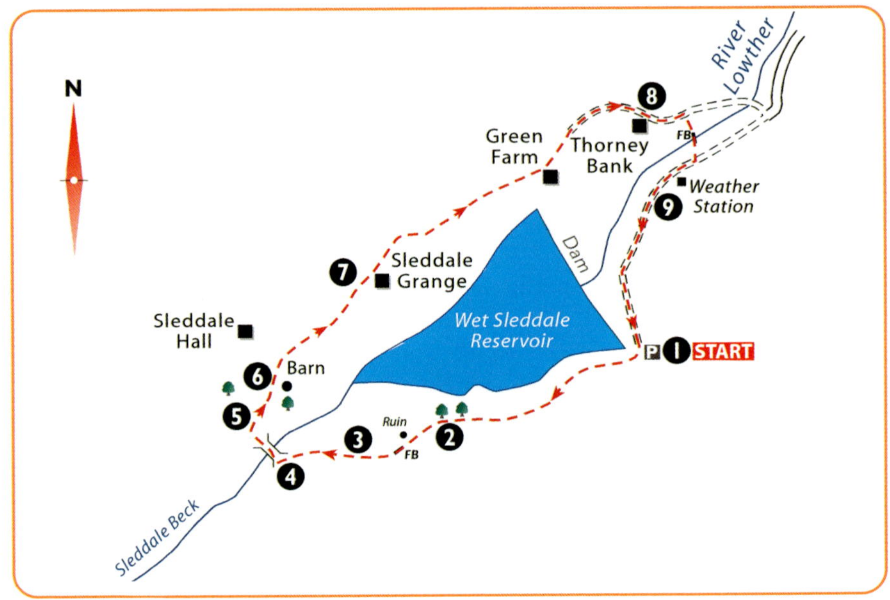

beside a stone wall. It then descends for a short distance and continues over undulating ground that can be boggy after rain. The reservoir is out of view at this point.

4. The path is not very clear for a while, but several white-topped marker posts help to keep you on track. Pass through a gap in another wall and then descend slightly to the right until you reach a wooden gate and a stone bridge which spans the Sleddale Beck.

This bridge featured in the film Withnail and I. *Underneath its arch are interesting stalactites, which have formed from the mortar used to construct the bridge.*

5. Having crossed the bridge, continue up the hillside, following the marker posts with white arrows and ignoring the path which goes right, just after the bridge. Climb the hillside and you will soon reach a wooden single step stile, which you cross. Then turn right and proceed up the track which rises up the hillside. Carry on through a wooded area.

6. You will reach a junction in the path with a substantial barn on your right. On the hillside above you is Wet Sleddale Hall. Bear right and follow the footpath sign on the stone wall, which directs you through a wooden gate and past the barn. Just after the barn are some small boulders which make convenient seats for a break.

7. Proceed along the main track. You will come to farm buildings at Sleddale Grange. Continue through

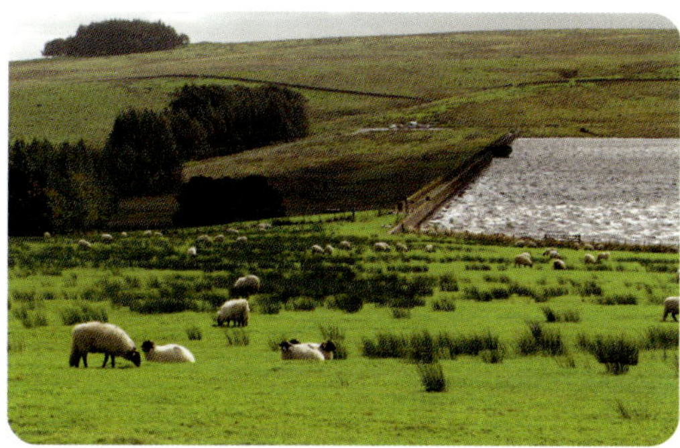

The dam wall seen across the fields

the yard. Your route descends through a metal gate, passing modern barns. Go through another metal gate and meet a tarmac road. Follow this road as it descends past Green Farm. Carry on along the track and go through a metal gate onto a minor road.

8. Proceed down the road, ignoring the high step stile over the wall on your right. As you reach another farm at Thorney Bank, you might see the Victorian postbox inset into the wall, near the entrance. The road runs next to the River Lowther for a short distance. Look for the elegant arched wooden footbridge that crosses the river on your right. Cross the river here. Join the road and then turn right. Proceed along the road in the general direction of the dam. On your left, you will soon pass a Met Office weather station, which is protected by a high fence. Continue over a cattle grid and past more farm buildings.

9. Continue along the road, passing another cattle grid.

There are close-up views of the dam wall along this section of the walk. When the water level is high the overflow can be a spectacular sight.

Make your way along the road, which now bends to the left and then rises up towards the car park where you started your walk.

NEARBY ATTRACTIONS

The remains of **Shap Abbey** are located approximately half a mile west of Shap, beside the River Lowther. The **Greyhound Hotel**, Shap, telephone: 01931 716474.

ST BEES

It is a good idea to take binoculars with you on this walk. The route follows a cliff-top track along St Bees Head, passing spectacular colonies of sea birds. You might also see harbour porpoise, which often swim just off the headland. Your route passes beside an attractive lighthouse, and then takes a short diversion through farmland before rejoining the coastal path.

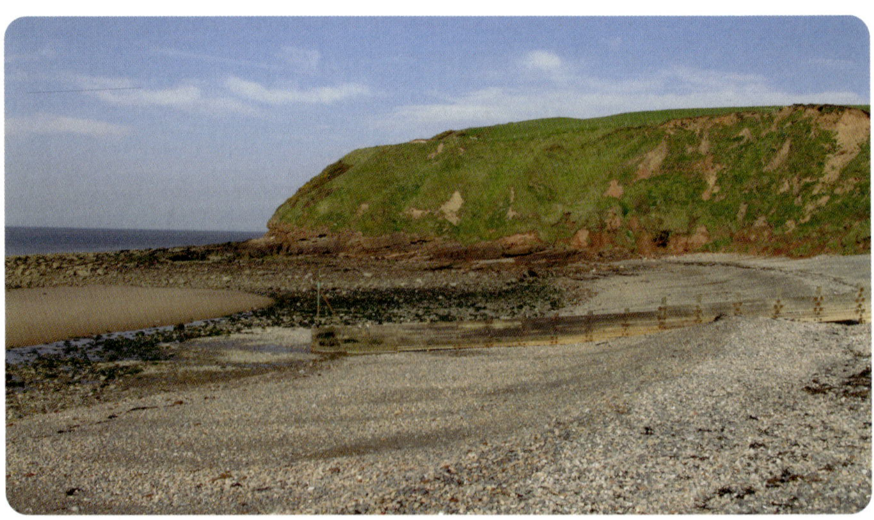

St Bees Head from the beach

- **HOW TO GET THERE:** From Whitehaven follow the B5345. Continue through St Bees for just over half a mile until you reach the car park below South Head.
- **PARKING:** The large pay-and-display car park by the sea shore.
- **LENGTH OF THE WALK:** 4.8 miles/7.8 kilometres. **MAP:** OS Explorer 303, (GR NX 961118).
- **TERRAIN:** A short uphill section, followed by easy walking along grassy paths. Extra care should to be taken when walking along the cliff top. Young children should be closely supervised. The many stiles along the route make it very difficult to take along all but the smallest of dogs.

St Bees is situated on the coast of Cumbria. The village is named after St Bega, whose life and miracles are described in the 13th-century text *Life of St Bega*. The author of *Life of St Bega* believed that she was an Irish king's daughter who valued virginity. When she was promised in marriage to a Viking prince 'son of the King of Norway', she fled across the Irish Sea and landed in this remote spot on the Cumbrian coast, where she settled and led a life of piety. Then, fearing the raids of pirates, which were occurring along the coast, she moved to Northumbria.

Your route along the top of St Bees Head passes nationally important bird colonies. The sights and sounds are extraordinary. Thousands of birds, including guillemots, kittiwakes, fulmars and razorbills, nest on the cliffs. Ravens and peregrine falcons are often seen skimming along the cliff tops and offshore you can also spot skuas and shearwaters. If you are lucky, you might spot dolphins and porpoises.

THE WALK

1. From the car park, walk towards the shore; then immediately turn right. Follow the top of the grassy bank or the concrete walkway along the line of the fence which borders the caravan park.

2. Cross the wooden footbridge over the small stream and follow the rough, sandy path uphill, towards the top of the cliff. (Ignore the footpath which branches right for Rottington.)

3. Continue on the undulating path that follows the cliff top. You should start to see the St Bees lighthouse in the distance. The path now descends down a series of steps into a small gorge, which leads into Fleswick Bay. Then, climb the path on the other side of the gorge, up a series of steps, which leads you back onto the headland.

4. Follow the path (a little faint at first) along the grassy top which runs parallel to the fence. You will soon reach the first of two viewpoints where you can observe the colonies of birds, which nest precariously on the cliff edges. The viewpoint is reached by means of a small stile over the fence on your left.

5. Rejoin the path and follow it until you see another viewpoint on your left, then carry on until you reach St Bees lighthouse.

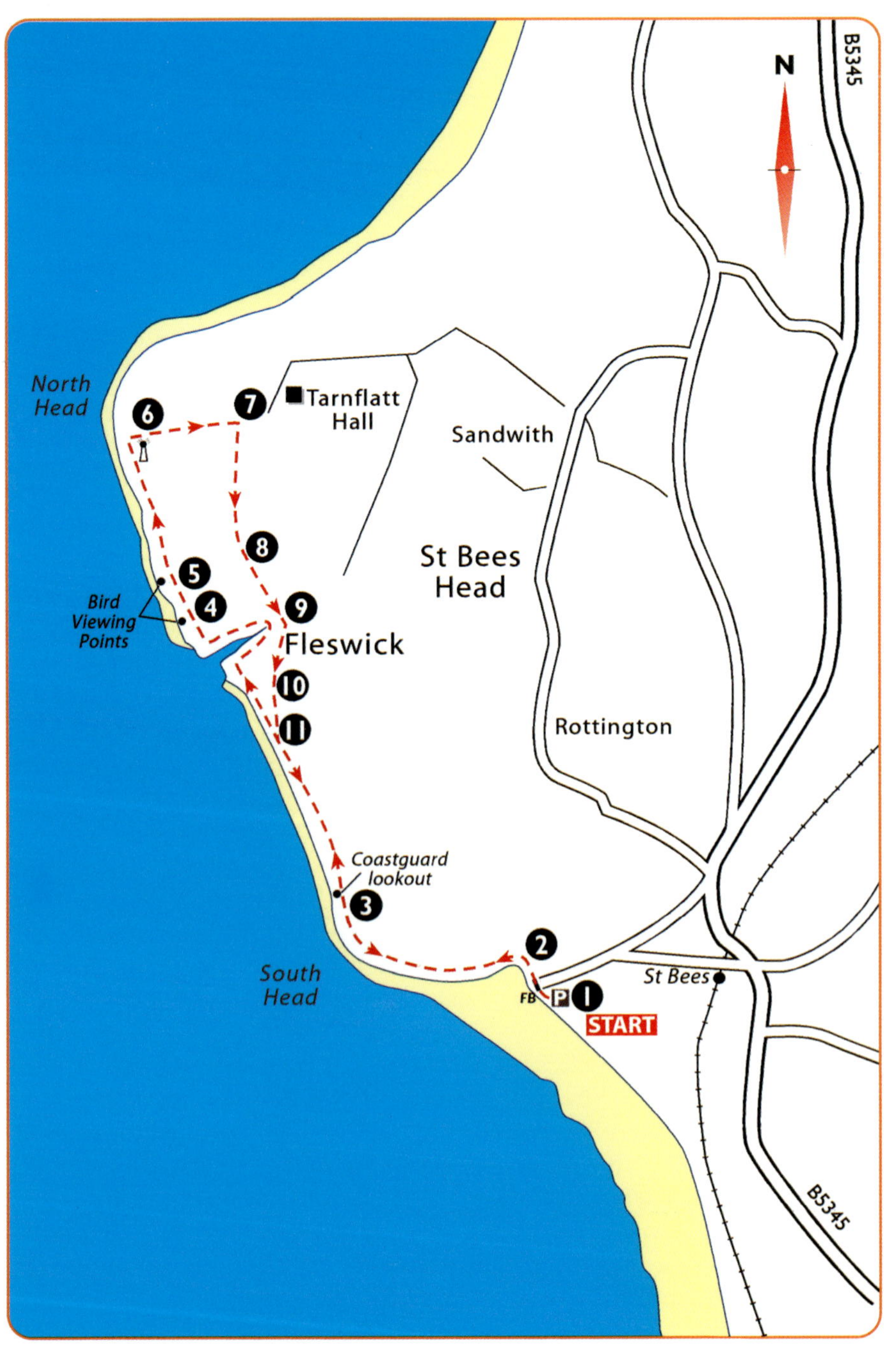

N
B5345
North Head
Tarnflatt Hall
Sandwith
St Bees Head
Bird Viewing Points
Rottington
Fleswick
Coastguard lookout
South Head
St Bees
FB
START
B5345

This 17-metre lighthouse was built in 1822. It replaced the original lighthouse, constructed in 1718, which was destroyed by fire. The lighthouse was de-manned in 1987 and is monitored from an operations control centre in Harwich. Every 20 seconds, its 1500 watt lamp beams two flashes, with an intensity of 134,000 candela, over a range of 21 nautical miles.

6. Leave the coastal path at this point by turning right, immediately before a fence and stile that leads to a white building on the cliff top. You will now pass beside the lighthouse, go through a kissing gate and continue down a road.

7. Walk down the road for approximately 400 metres. Look for a stile next to a metal gate and a small sign on your right, inscribed: 'DEFRA conservation walks'. Leave the road here and take the path through the field.

8. Carry on through several fields, walking alongside the field boundaries on your left. The path is occasionally obscure. You might see the sea in the distance ahead of you. Your route now descends and emerges at the tip of the small gorge which leads to Fleswick Bay. (You crossed through this gorge earlier.)

9. Bear slightly left, along a rough track, keeping the start of the gorge over to your right.

10. Keep straight on, and then descend gradually to your right, through fields, on a faint path which leads back onto the coastal path. You are now back on the cliff-top path along which you travelled earlier.

11. Turn left here, keeping the sea on your right, and return along your original route towards the beach at St Bees.

NEARBY ATTRACTIONS
St Bees village, including **The Priory**, the old school and the birthplace of Edmund Grindal. **The Seacote Hotel**, The Beach, St Bees, telephone: 01946 822300.

WAST WATER

This route is a classic Lake District walk, which circumnavigates Wast Water, the deepest body of water in the Lake District. The landscape is magnificent throughout, and the scenery at the head of the valley has been voted 'Britain's Favourite View'.

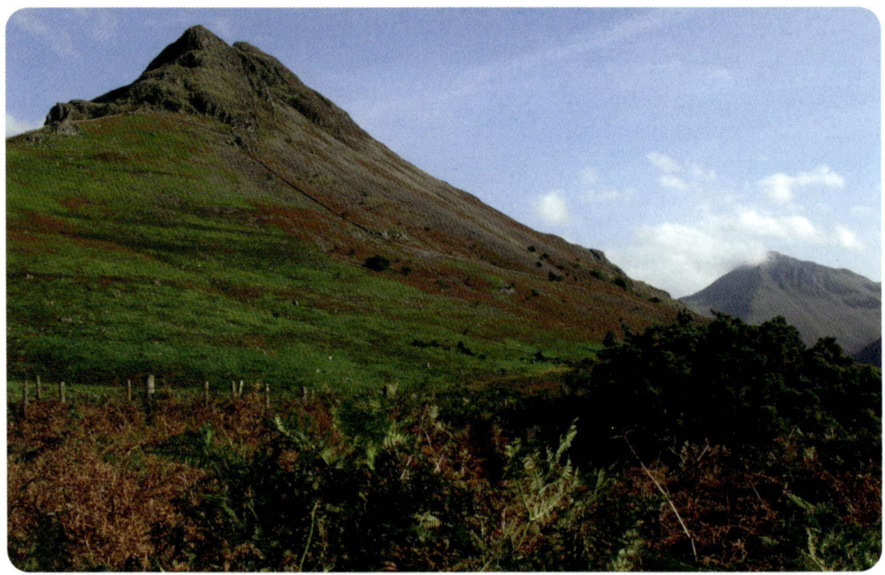

Yewbarrow can be seen at point 1 of the route

- **HOW TO GET THERE:** From the A595 follow the signs for Wasdale. When you reach the road beside Wast Water, follow signs to Wasdale Head. Continue along the lakeshore road to a car park.
- **PARKING:** The National Trust car park at Overbeck Bridge, on the western shore of Wast Water.
- **LENGTH OF THE WALK:** 7.9 miles/12.7 kilometres. **MAP:** OS Explorer OL6 (GR NY 168068).
- **TERRAIN:** There is an arduous section of scree where extra care and concentration are needed. The section of scree makes it difficult to take dogs on this walk.

Your route does a circuit of Wast Water. The lake is three miles long and half a mile wide. With a depth of 80 metres (263 ft), it is the deepest body of water in the Lake District. Its depth and clear water make it popular with divers. The lake was the scene of a murder investigation in 1984, when divers discovered the body of the 'Wasdale Lady in the Lake'; she had been murdered eight years earlier and her body disposed of in the lake. The body settled at a depth of 34 metres (110 ft), only a short distance away from a much deeper part of the lake, where it might never have been found. The victim's husband later confessed to her murder.

The rock-littered slopes on the south-eastern side of the lake that lead up to the summits of Illgill Head and Whin Rigg are known as the Wast Water Screes. The screes resulted from the erosion of the rocks of the Borrowdale volcanic group, that form the fells on this side of the lake. They are one of the best and most famous examples of screes in Britain, and they are constantly on the move.

In 1815, Louis Simond, in his book *Journal of a Tour and Residence of Great Britain* recalled a spectacular event which had occurred a few years earlier: 'scaling of the rocks over Wast-Water produced a sort of continued avalanche of stones for some weeks, raising a promontory into the lake … a column of dust was observable for some miles rising in the air over the spot.'

THE WALK

1. From the car park, turn left and walk along the road towards Wasdale Head, keeping the lake on your right.

The angular peak that you can see rising up on your left is Yewbarrow. In the distance, at the head of the valley, is Great Gable, and across the lake to your half-right is the Scafell massif.

As you reach the end of the lake, cross over a cattle grid and continue ahead. Ignore the step stile through the wall and carry on along the road.

2. You will reach a right turn signed for Wasdale camp site, with a wooden fingerpost indicating 'public footpath Scafell Massif, Eskdale'. Turn right here and continue down the side road. Cross the bridge over Lingmell Beck. The beck is a rare spawning ground for the threatened Arctic charr. Proceed down the track, passing the camp site and a car park on your left. Continue over the cattle grid and then over another bridge. Follow the track which bears right towards the lake. A wooden

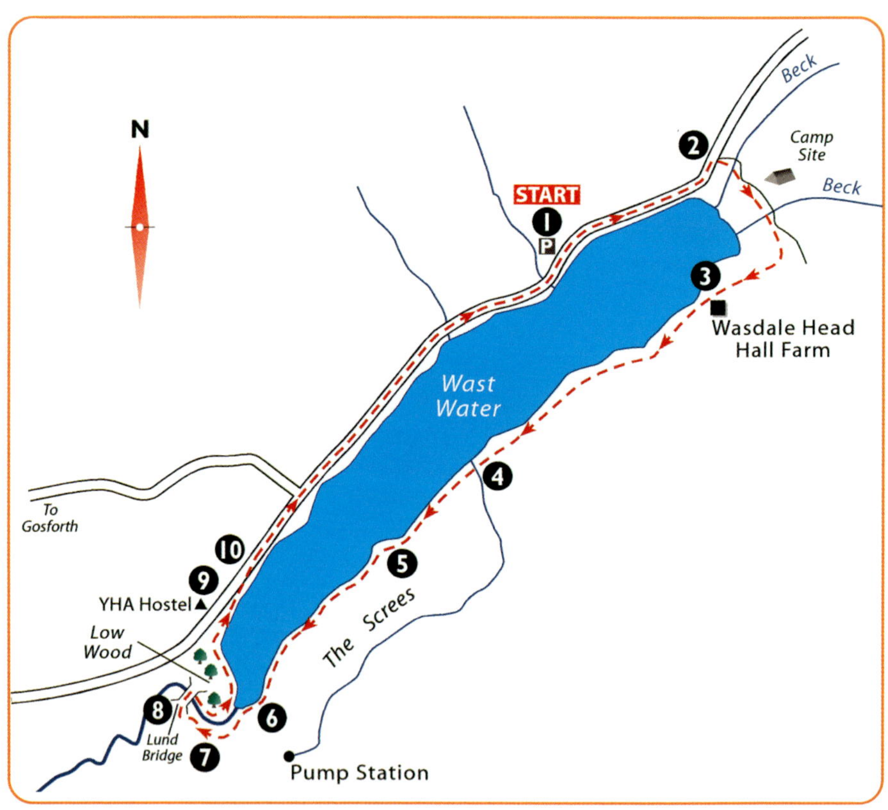

fingerpost directs you to the lake shore. Follow the farm track which leads towards Wasdale Head Hall Farm.

3. Just before you reach the entrance to the farm, go through the wooden gate directly in front of you. Continue through the field, keeping the lake to your right and the farm over to your left. Go through a wooden gate and then reach another, which displays a warning notice about the screes. Proceed through a gap in a wall and continue along a rough, bracken-fringed path. The route narrows and ascends slightly, and then begins to traverse the steeply-angled fellside.

4. You will reach the start of several sections of scree. At this point, the scree consists of small pieces of rock, and you might wonder what all the fuss is about. However, it becomes boulder-sized later on. Make your way along the foot-worn shelf that traverses the steep scree slope. The

60

lake is close by on your right, and you can peer down into its deep water. Proceed over several grassy sections before reaching more continuous stretches of scree.

5. You will arrive at a small cluster of silver birch trees and a couple of small oak trees. Ahead of you is one of the toughest sections of scree. There are continuous stretches of large boulders with no obvious paths across them. Occasionally, small piles of rocks are placed to act as mini cairns to guide your way.

Stow away any walking poles so you can use your hands for extra balance. Be aware that boulders can shift under your weight. Take it slowly and concentrate. Rest often and remember to admire the views!

A short section of path offers some respite, and then you are back onto another section of boulders. Press on; it starts to get easier.

6. You will start to approach the end of the lake. Ahead of you, in the middle distance, is a stone building. Conditions underfoot now become easier as the scree becomes finer. Your route descends towards the stone building. This is Wast Water pump house, which stands next to a shallow bay, near an attractive boathouse. The River Irt runs out of Wast Water here.

7. Continue down the track, keeping the River Irt on your right. You will be relieved to be walking along an easy track after your recent exertions. Pass through a wooden kissing gate next to a metal gate, and then continue for a few metres until you see another kissing gate on your right. Leave the track through the kissing gate and go onto a narrow path which leads through a wooded area beside the River Irt. Follow the path beside the river, passing through two more kissing gates.

8. You will arrive at a lovely stone bridge, known as Lund Bridge. Cross the river at this point, and then go through a wooden gate before bearing right, through a kissing gate which leads into Low Wood. In the wood you are faced with a fork in the path. Keep right, following the general course of the river, which is now on your right. You will soon reach the shore of the pretty bay that you saw earlier, from the opposite side. Continue along the path until you reach a junction in front of a grassy knoll covered with trees. Go right here and head towards the boathouse.

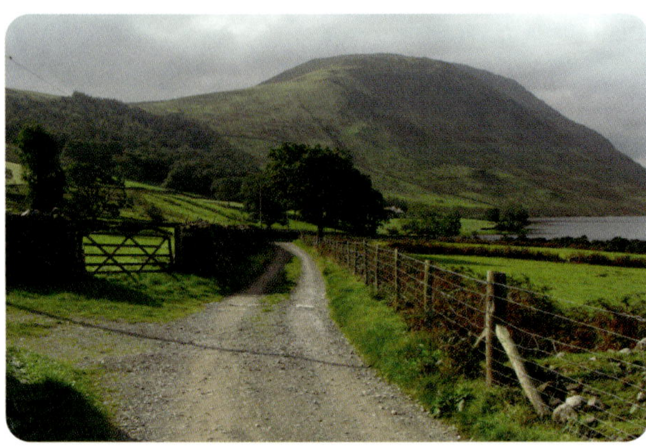

*The track to Wasdale
Head Hall Farm*

Your route passes behind the boathouse and then bears left. Continue along the path, with the lake shore on your right.

9. Carry on through a wooden gate and leave the wood. Follow the lake shore path. Over to your left, you will see a large building with a mock-Tudor frontage. This is Wast Water Youth Hostel, which dates from 1829 and is owned by the National Trust. Make your way through a kissing gate into a field containing impressive oak trees. Go through another kissing gate (with an inscription on it) and proceed along a grassy section of path.

10. Your route now goes through a cluster of rhododendrons. You will soon reach a series of stone steps and a high wooden step-stile that takes you over a wall. Climb the stile and continue to follow the path for a few metres until you reach the road. Turn right here, towards Wasdale Head. The last section of your walk follows the quiet lake shore road for 1.85 miles/2.9 kilometres back to your starting point. Along the way you can admire 'Britain's Favourite View'.

NEARBY ATTRACTIONS

The **Wasdale Head Inn** (telephone: 01946 726229) is situated at the head of remote and unspoiled Wasdale. The Great Gable Brewing Company is located next to the pub and supplies it with a range of cask ales. **St Olaf's church** at Wasdale Head is one of England's smallest churches. The roof beams are thought to have come from Viking ships. In the churchyard are the graves of pioneering rock climbers who have died on the surrounding fells.

RYDAL WATER

This walk is steeped in literary history. En route you will pass Rydal Mount, once the home of William Wordsworth, and Nab Cottage, which was formerly Thomas de Quincey's residence. The first part of your route follows an old coffin track, and then passes Dora's Field, a spectacular sight in spring when the daffodils are in bloom. You continue beside Rydal Water and finish with a stroll alongside the pretty River Rothay.

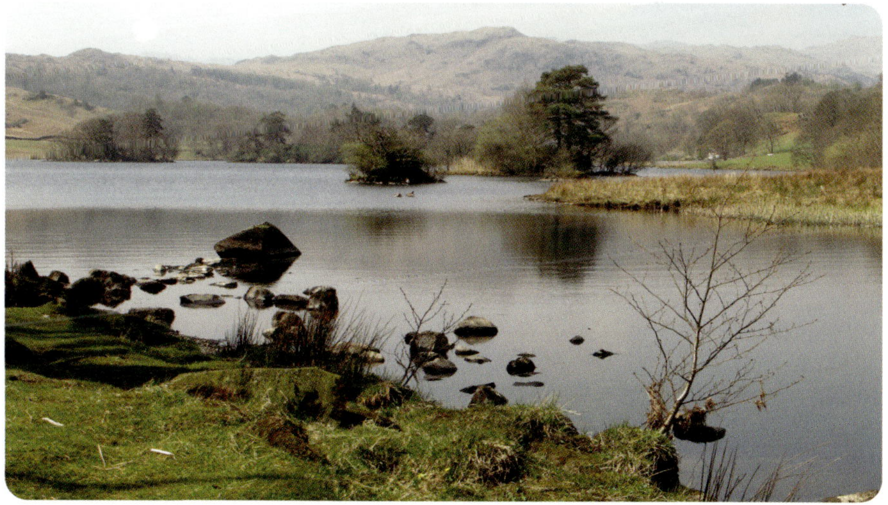

The beautiful Rydal Water

- **HOW TO GET THERE:** From Ambleside follow the A591 towards Grasmere. The road follows the side of Rydal Water for a while. As you reach the end of the lake, turn right into White Moss car park.
- **PARKING:** White Moss car park (pay-and-display).
- **LENGTH OF THE WALK:** 3.4 miles/5.4 kilometres. **MAP:** OS Explorer OL7 (GR NY 349065).
- **TERRAIN:** A short climb is followed by a walk along rough undulating paths. The paths are generally easy to follow. Care is needed on the short section of road beside Rydal Mount, as there is no pavement.

Rydal Mount was the home of William Wordsworth and his family from 1813 to 1850. They rented the house from Lady le Fleming, of nearby Rydal Hall. The poet composed and revised many of his poems here, including his famous *Daffodils*, which was published in 1815. Wordsworth died at Rydal Mount on 23rd April 1850.

The nearby church, St Mary's, dates from 1824. The site was originally an orchard owned by Lady le Fleming. Wordsworth helped choose the site for the church and was a churchwarden from 1833–1834. Next to the church is Dora's Field, which was once owned by Wordsworth. He had planned to build a house here. When Dora, his daughter, died in 1847, the heartbroken poet planted the hillside with daffodils in her memory. In early spring the field is a blaze of yellow daffodils, which are later replaced by a carpet of bluebells. Dora's Field is now owned by the National Trust.

Your route continues alongside beautiful Rydal Water. The lake was formerly known as Routhmere, named after the River Rothay, which drains from it. *Rothay* is derived from Old Scandinavian for 'trout river'.

On the roadside beside the lake is Nab Cottage, where the author and critic Thomas de Quincey lived. De Quincey wrote *Confessions of an English Opium-Eater*, an autobiographical account of his laudanum addiction and its effect on his life. The Confessions were first published anonymously in September and October 1821 in the *London Magazine* and were later released in book form in 1822. Its publication won him almost instant fame. By 1833, de Quincey, struggling with his opium addiction and financial troubles, was forced to leave Nab Cottage.

THE WALK

1. From White Moss car park, turn left along the side of the A591, towards Ambleside. Ignore the first footpath sign and take the next path on the left, just after a postbox. This path follows the stream uphill for a short distance. Just after a small waterfall, the path forks. A less distinct track leads off to the left. Keep to the more obvious path on the right, which ascends the hillside between two drystone walls.

2. After a short climb, you will reach a T-junction in the path. Turn right here and follow the path that traverses the hillside. At this point, you will see Rydal Water on your right and Loughrigg Fell, which stands behind it.

3. Follow this track as it undulates along the base of Nab Scar. This route

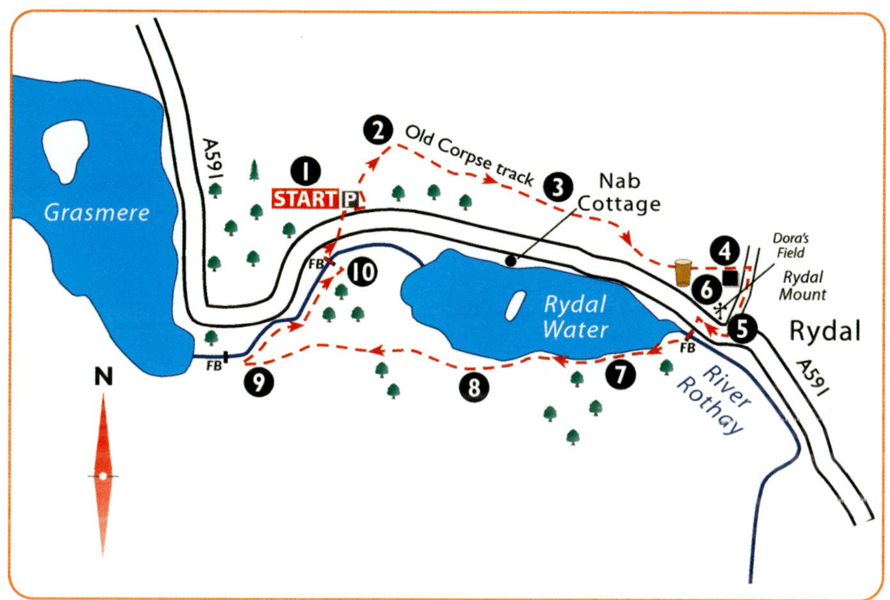

is known as a coffin track, because, until Rydal was granted its parish status, coffins were carried along this route to the church in Grasmere.

As you follow the path, you may see a white house on the roadside to your right. This is Nab Cottage, originally built in 1556 as a simple farmstead, and rebuilt in 1702. Between 1817 and 1833 it was the home of Thomas de Quincey.

4. Your route gradually descends into a small hamlet. Over the wall, on your right, you will see the impressive chimneystacks of Rydal Mount. Turn right and descend along the road in front of Rydal Mount.

5. Continue down the road. As you approach the main road, you will pass St Mary's, on your right, with its attractive churchyard. When you meet the main road (A591), turn right. Keep to the pavement. As you pass the church, you will see a small gate into Dora's Field.

6. When you get to the Glen Rothay Hotel and Badger Bar (once a 17th-century coaching inn), cross over the road and cut through the gap in the wall. This path leads over a bridge which spans the River Rothay. Once over the bridge, turn right towards the lake, along the path that follows the river. You soon reach Rydal Water. The grassy area under the trees on the side of the lake is a relaxing place to take a break. There are good views of the lake and its two main islands: Little Isle on the left, and Heron Island on the right.

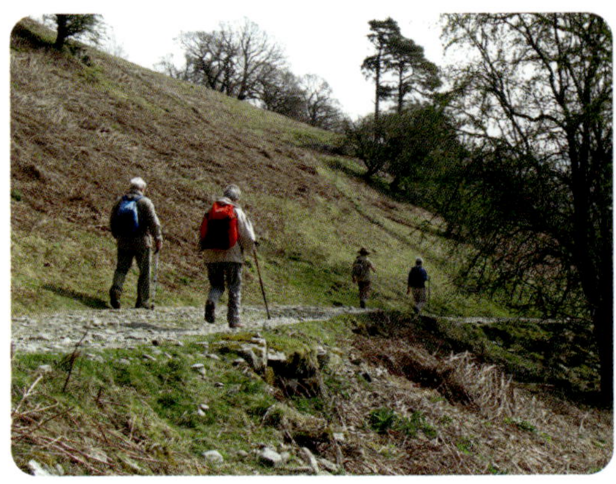

Walkers on the old 'coffin' track

7. Follow the lakeside path. The lake shore, with its lovely small bays, is a popular picnic spot in summer. On the opposite shore, you can see an attractive boathouse.

8. The path now leaves the side of the lake and climbs uphill, beside a stone wall. Continue on this main path, passing the ruin of an old farm building on your right. Ignore other paths that branch from it. Your path now zigzags up a short gradient. Once at the top, you can see both Grasmere and Rydal Water. Descend towards Grasmere. You will see a footbridge over the River Rothay, which flows from Grasmere.

9. Don't cross the footbridge; instead, turn right just before it. Then follow the river (on your left) downstream as it cuts through the woods in a series of small rapids and pools. Wild garlic grows along its shady banks.

10. When you reach a large wooden footbridge, cross over the river and proceed along the path, which bears right. Carry on until you reach a bend in the river. A path branches off to the left here, which takes you back to the A591 and the car park where you started your walk.

NEARBY ATTRACTIONS

Rydal Mount, the former home of William Wordsworth, is located close by and is open to the public. **Ambleside** is a bustling town with a wide range of shops, pubs, cafés and galleries. Ambleside Tourist Information Centre is based at Central Buildings, Market Cross, Ambleside, LA22 9BS, telephone: 01539 432583.

ELTER WATER AND LOUGHRIGG TARN

Starting from the 'chocolate box' village of Elterwater, your route climbs to reveal the famous mountains of the Langdale Pikes. You visit a beautiful, lily-fringed tarn, and then descend to the River Brathay to see its powerful waterfall, Skelwith Force. Your course then passes the banks of Elter Water before following Great Langdale Beck back to the village.

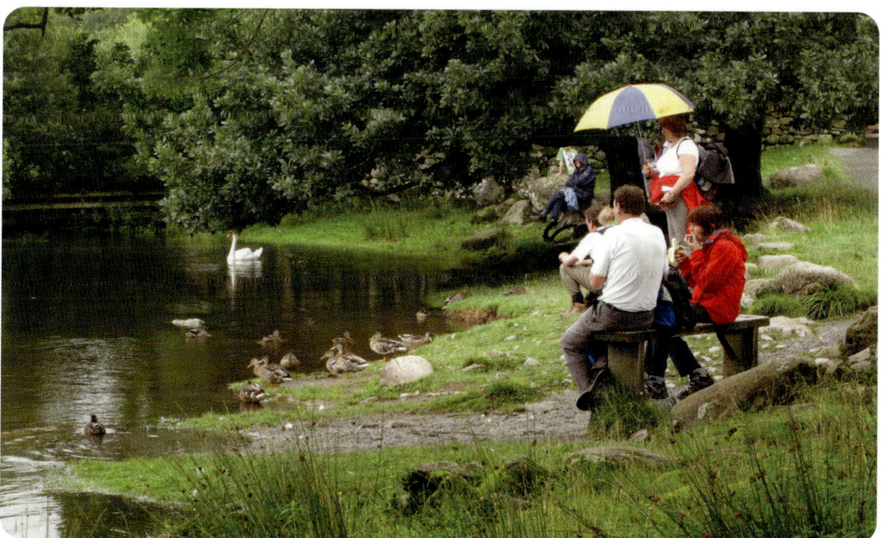

The shore of Elter Water

- **HOW TO GET THERE:** From Ambleside follow the A593, and then take the B5343. Leave the B5343 and descend into the centre of the village.
- **PARKING:** The National Trust pay-and-display car park beside the bridge.
- **LENGTH OF THE WALK:** 3.6 miles/5.8 kilometres. **MAP:** OS Explorer OL7 (GR NY 328047).
- **TERRAIN:** A gradual ascent along an obvious route, followed by an easy descent and then a final stretch of mostly level paths. You are advised to closely supervise young children and keep dogs on a lead when passing through the slate works and at Skelwith Force.

Elterwater village takes its name from the nearby lake, Elter Water, derived from the Old Scandinavian *eltr vatn* 'swan lake'. Swans have been migrating here for hundreds of years. The village has a green and a traditional Lake District pub, the Britannia, which is over 400-years-old and was a gentleman farmer's residence before becoming a coaching inn. The Britannia serves home-made food, fine wines and real ales.

The nearby Langdale complex was a 17th-century woollen mill, where local wool was processed using machinery driven by Great Langdale Beck. From 1823 the site was used as a gunpowder works, Elterwater Gunpowder Works developed with the growing demand for explosives from the region's mines and quarries. It also exported its produce to North America and South Africa. The gunpowder was stored in wooden barrels made at a cooper's shop in the village. The works closed in 1930, as a result of the Great Depression and the development of dynamite.

Your route passes Loughrigg Tarn, a picturesque little tarn fringed with water lilies, which nestles under Loughrigg Fell and has excellent views across to the Langdale Pikes. The tarn was used as a location for the Beatrix Potter movie. Wordsworth called Loughrigg Tarn 'Diana's looking glass'. He wrote

'Thus gladdened from our own dear vale we pass
And soon approach Diana's Looking-glass!
To Loughrigg-tarn, round clear and bright as heaven.'

THE WALK

1. Leave the car park and turn right. Follow the road which branches right, passing the bowling club and then the Judy Boyes Studio. Continue following the road uphill until you reach the main road (B5343). In the distance, on your left, you will see the famous mountains of Harrison Stickle, Pavey Ark and Pike 'O Stickle, known collectively as the Langdale Pikes. Turn right and follow the B5343 a short distance as it gradually climbs uphill and crosses a cattle grid. The road then descends slightly.

2. On your right you will soon see a stone house called **Guide Post**. Turn left here to follow the minor road opposite. A painted block of stone at the junction of this road displays distances to nearby villages. Continue along the road as it climbs uphill, passing a side road on your right.

3. When you reach a road junction, turn right and follow the road as it

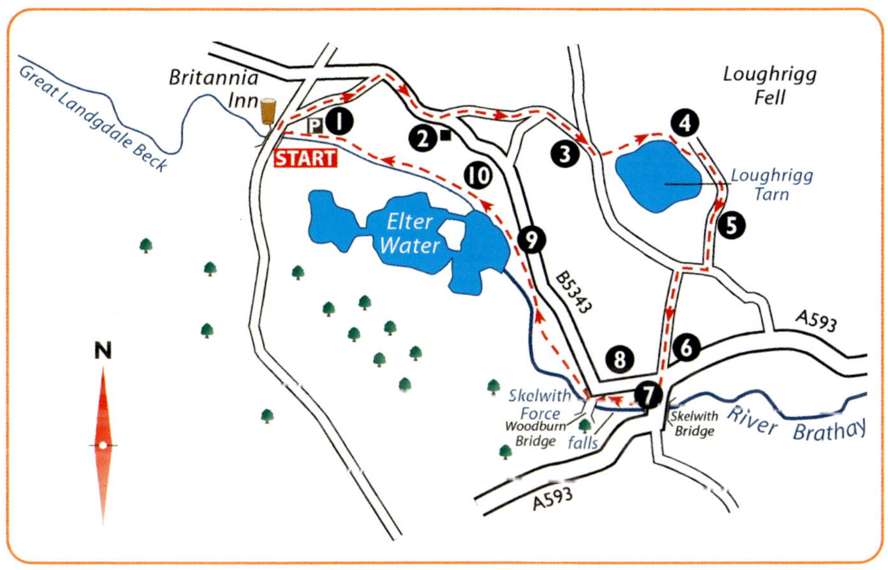

descends. Loughrigg Tarn will soon be revealed to your left. Watch for a gate and stile on your left. It is sometimes hidden behind cars which park in front of it. Leave the road here and climb over the stile, following the fingerpost through farm fields towards the tarn. Proceed through the first field and then climb a ladder stile over a stone wall.

4. Follow the path which skirts the edge of the tarn. This is a beautiful setting and the tarn is popular with fishermen and picnickers. You may spot a small wooden cross near the water's edge, a memorial to John Stanley Skelton, who drowned here in 1960. Continue along the path and then locate a gate through the iron fence ahead of you, which takes you onto a farm track. Turn right and follow the track. You will pass a small campsite on your right.

5. You will soon reach a wooden gate next to Tarn Foot Lodge. Pass through the gate, and keep straight ahead, along the track. Ignore the footpath to Ambleside on your left. Descend until you reach a minor road. Turn right and follow this road until you reach a stream that passes under the road, with a road junction on your left. Turn left here and continue down the minor road. The road descends through a wooded area, passing Oak Dene, a single storey stone building on your left, and the entrance to Neaum Crag on your right.

6. The road steepens and makes an S-bend before meeting the major road junction next to the Skelwith Bridge Hotel. Cross over the B5343 (on your right) and then follow the A593 for 100 metres, passing the Skelwith Bridge Hotel. Turn right immediately before the road bridge. You will see a fingerpost: 'public footpath Elterwater'. Follow this sign. On your right is an attractive row of cottages with unusual chimney stacks.

7. Your route now follows the track which forks right. Follow the sign for 'deliveries and footpath' in front of several slate slabs that are set into the ground. Continue through the Kirkstone Quarries slate works.

8. Carry on into the woods beside the River Brathay.

You will soon reach Skelwith Force waterfall. If you want a closer look, a couple of small bridges lead to viewing points overlooking the falls.

Proceed along the path and pass Woodburn Bridge, a beautifully designed, elegant modern bridge, which crosses the river. Keep straight on; don't cross the bridge.

9. Go through a narrow kissing gate to emerge from the woods into open fields. Follow this level, easy section of footpath. The craggy mountains provide a magnificent backdrop here, and the river, with it deep glides, is particularly picturesque at this point. Make your way along the path until you reach the end of Elter Water Lake. You might spot some of the lake's swans here. Go through a gate into another section of woodland. Stick to the main track.

10. After a while, your route joins the edge of a shallow, gravel-bottomed river. This is Great Langdale Beck. Continue along the path that follows the riverbank. You will see Elterwater village ahead of you. Continue until you reach a wooden gate near the road bridge over the river. Your start point is on your right.

NEARBY ATTRACTIONS

Ambleside is a bustling town with a wide range of shops, pubs, cafés and galleries. Ambleside Tourist Information Centre is based at Central Buildings, Market Cross, Ambleside, LA22 9BS, telephone: 015394 32 583. The **Britannia Inn**, Elterwater, telephone: 015394 37210.

RAVENGLASS

Your walk starts from the historic village of Ravenglass and passes a Roman bathhouse and the site of a Roman fort. The trail continues through secluded woodland beside the River Esk before emerging onto the estuary shore. The walk finishes with a stroll through the historic village, with a chance to uncover more of its fascinating past.

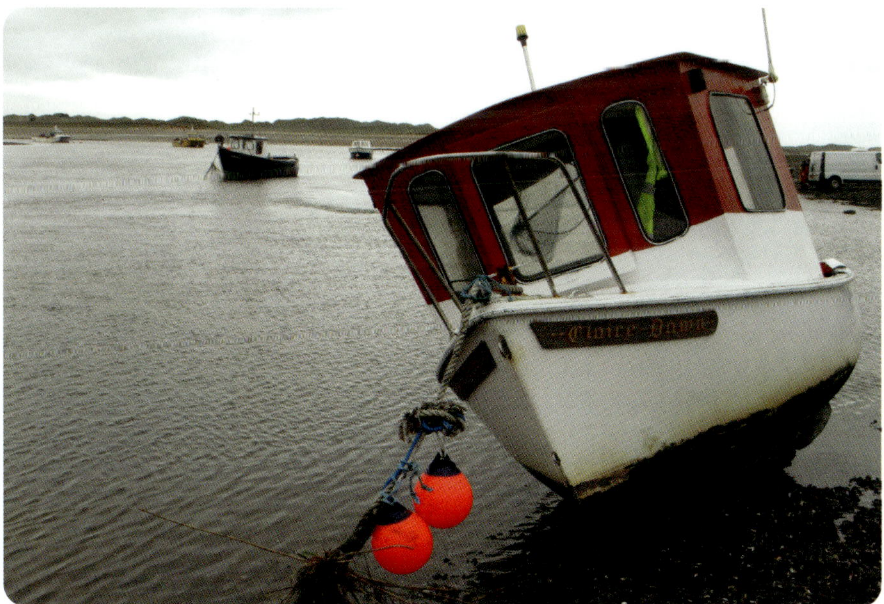

The estuary at Ravenglass

- **HOW TO GET THERE:** Leave the A595, following the sign for Ravenglass, and travel half a mile into the village.
- **PARKING:** The large free car park located just off Main Street.
- **LENGTH OF THE WALK:** 3.3 miles/5.3 kilometres. **MAP:** OS Explorer OL6. (GR SD 085964).
- **TERRAIN:** Generally, the going is easy and is mainly flat apart from one short uphill section. The path at the foot of Newtown Knott can be very muddy after wet weather.

Ravenglass is a coastal hamlet in the Lake District National Park. It lies on the estuary of three rivers: the Esk, the Mite and the Irt. An important Roman naval base in the 2nd century, it was known as *Glannoventa*. The base was a regional supply point for much of the north-west, and a road ran from Ravenglass through Hard Knott Pass to the Roman fort at Ambleside. Glannoventa had a garrison of 1,000 soldiers and was occupied for 300 years.

The fort was established around AD 130 on the site of a smaller fortlet built a decade earlier. Its defences were originally turf and timber but a stone wall was constructed early in the 3rd century. Today, all that remains of the main fort are some faint earthworks, but the nearby bathhouse is much better preserved and its 13-ft high walls are among the tallest Roman structures surviving in northern Britain.

THE WALK

1. Leave the car park at its rear exit, on the right-hand side. Follow the wooden fingerpost for the Roman bathhouse. A tarmac path leads you up between metal railings and then over a railway bridge. Continue down the path until you reach a gate and a road. Turn right here and follow the road. A wooden fingerpost directs you to the Roman bathhouse and Newtown Knott. Continue past the Ravenglass Camping and Caravanning Club site, on your left. Follow the path on the left, which runs parallel to the road.

2. You will soon reach the Roman bathhouse on your left.

In the field opposite you can see the raised earthworks of the Roman fort that stood here. An information board tells you more about its history.

3. Proceed along the footpath at the side of the road until you reach a fork in the road. A sign directs you to Knottview and Newtown. Bear left here and follow the wide track, which ascends gradually, through a wooded area. Stick to the main track, ignoring paths which branch from it. Continue up the track, keeping Newtown House and Knottview Cottage on your right.

4. The track bends to the right and passes barns at the back of the two houses. An old metal gate leads you onto a rough track with a stone wall on your right. Continue along the track and through another metal gate, which is flanked by two substantial stone gateposts.

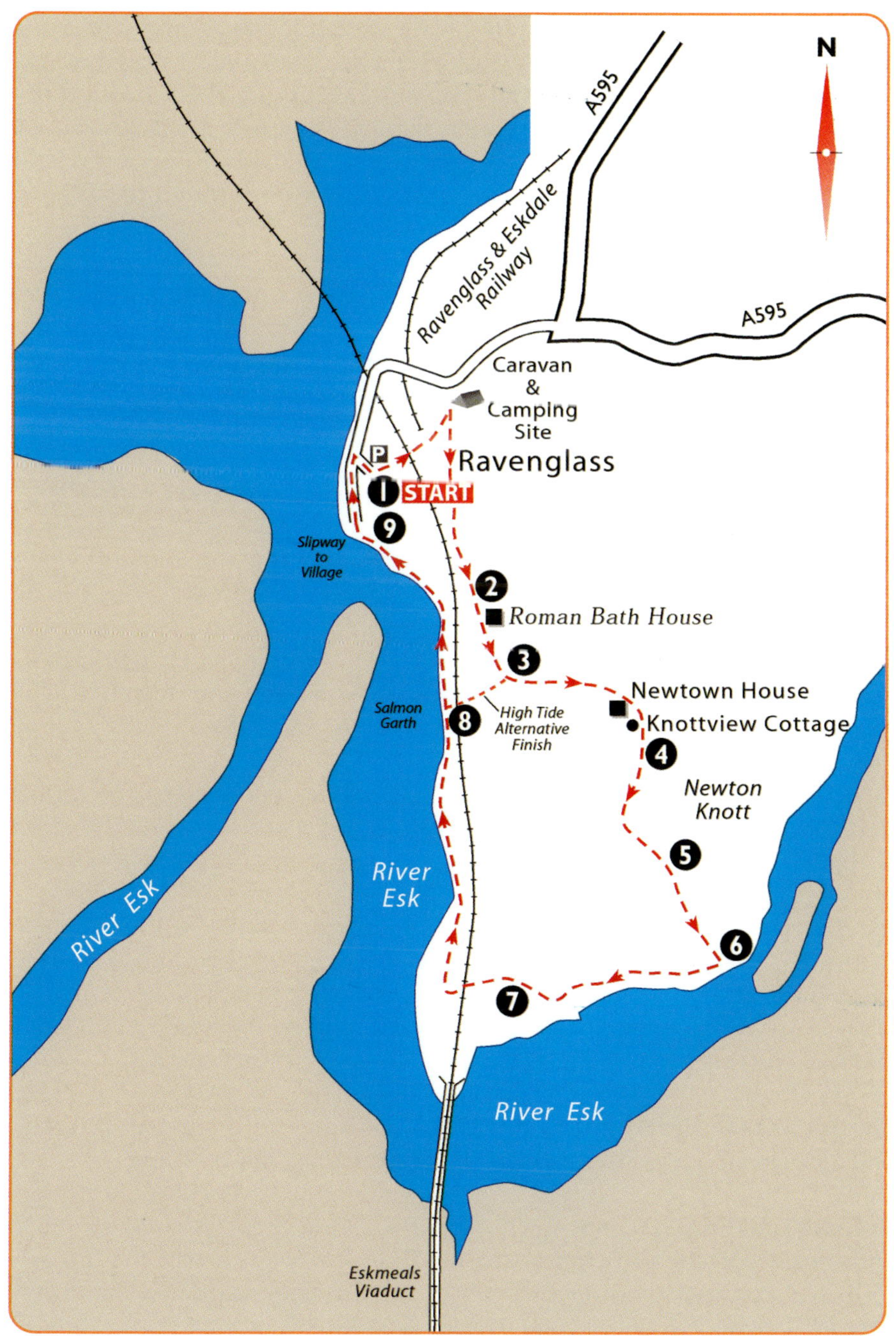
N
A595
A595
Ravenglass & Eskdale Railway
Caravan & Camping Site
Ravenglass
P
START
1
9
Slipway to Village
2
Roman Bath House
3
Newtown House
Knottview Cottage
4
8
High Tide Alternative Finish
Salmon Garth
Newton Knott
5
6
River Esk
River Esk
7
River Esk
Eskmeals Viaduct

5. Ascend the (sometimes muddy) track until it levels off and you reach a faint junction. Bear right here, just after a low, rocky knoll, and descend through a gate in the stone wall. You should see the river through the trees ahead of you. Descend through the field, towards the river. Several white-topped wooden posts mark your route. At the bottom of the field you will reach a gate and a kissing gate. Continue through the kissing gate into a wooded area.

6. A narrow path runs through the trees. When you reach a T-junction in the path, with the River Esk in front of you, turn right and follow the path through a secluded section of woodland. The Esk is visible on your left as it flows downstream towards the Ravenglass estuary. Your route then winds through the woods until you reach a dilapidated wooden gate through a stone wall. Go through the gate, passing blackthorn trees. Their fruits, sloes, can be used to make sloe gin.

7. You now reach an open area with salt marsh on your left and views across to the Eskmeals viaduct. Carry on along the path that runs beside the edge of the marsh towards the railway embankment. Go under the small bridge and then through a wooden gate. You now get views across the estuary. Continue ahead, following the path along the shoreline. The houses that you can see in the distance are in Ravenglass.

The shoreline and the exposed sand banks are good places to spot a wide variety of wading birds. At low tide the wooden posts of the old salmon garth can also be seen, once used to string out fishing nets.

8. There are alternative finishing routes for this walk. At low tide the shoreline path can be followed all the way back to the village. At high tide, leave the shoreline path by taking the track which bears right and passes under the railway line. Then, turn left along the road to reach the Roman bathhouse, and then retrace your steps to the car park.

9. If you take the low tide route you will ascend a slipway into the village. This is Main Street, lined with interesting old buildings.

NEARBY ATTRACTIONS
Take a ride on the **Ravenglass to Eskdale Railway** or visit the historic **Muncaster Castle** with its owl centre and attractive gardens. The **Ratty Arms**, Ravenglass, telephone: 01229 717676.

KELLY HALL TARN AND CONISTON WATER

This is a walk of two halves. The first part of your journey takes you across Torver Back Common, passing a photogenic little tarn, and across sparse, undulating terrain. The second part takes you through peaceful woodland and then along a quiet trail beside Coniston Water.

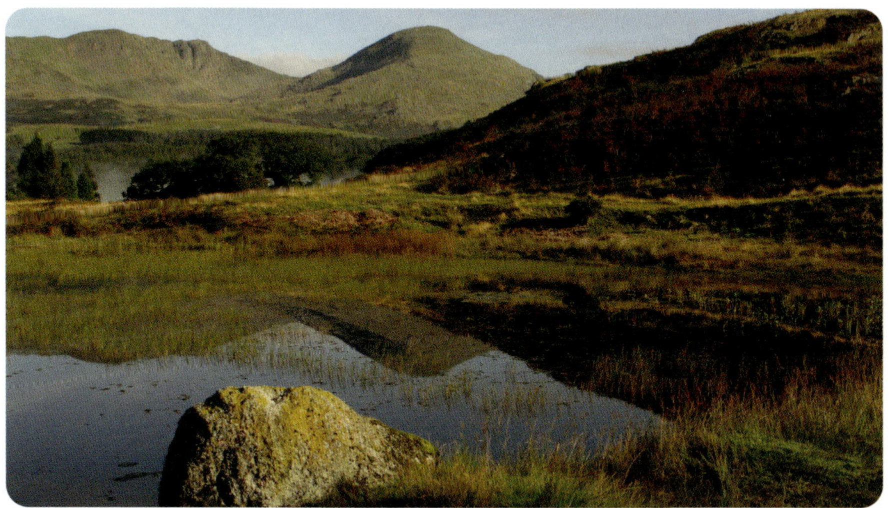

Looking towards the Old Man of Coniston from Kelly Hall Tarn

- **HOW TO GET THERE:** The village of Torver is located approximately 2.5 miles south of the town of Coniston, on the A593. Your starting point is situated at Beckstones, just off the B5084, about ¾ mile south of Torver.
- **PARKING:** An area of rough ground opposite the Lakeland Land Rover garage at Beckstones. Another parking area, located down the road from here, has space for a similar number of vehicles.
- **LENGTH OF THE WALK:** 3.4 miles/5.5 kilometres. **MAP:** OS Explorer OL6 (GR SD 287931).
- **TERRAIN:** Rough paths. The path across Torver Common is a little indistinct and can be difficult to see in poor visibility or when there is snow on the ground.

Torver is a small hamlet just over 2 miles south-west of Coniston village. It was originally a Norse settlement and the name Torver comes from Scandinavian *torf* 'turf'. Between the village and Coniston Water lies Torver Back Common with its pretty tarns. Kelly Hall Tarn is particularly beautiful and is said to have been named after a nearby building that has since been demolished.

The second half of your walk takes you alongside Coniston Water. The lake has become identified with the dramatic death of Donald Campbell, who was trying to set a new world water speed record in his jet-powered boat *Bluebird*. He set off down the lake on 4th January 1967 and achieved a run of 297 mph on his first leg. He then turned around without waiting for his wake to settle, and set off on his second leg. Shortly after passing Peel Island, exceeding a speed of 300 mph, *Bluebird* lifted out of the water, somersaulted and disintegrated upon hitting the water's surface. Campbell's last words on his final run were recorded via his radio intercom:

'Pitching a bit down here...Probably from my own wash...Straightening up now on track...Rather close to Peel Island...Tramping like mad... Full power...Tramping like hell here... I can't see much... and the water's very bad indeed...I can't get over the top... I'm getting a lot of bloody row in here... I can't see anything... I've got the bows up... I've gone...oh.'

THE WALK

1. From the parking area opposite the Land Rover garage, go up the rough track which heads away from the road. Continue through a kissing gate next to a large wooden gate. Pass a sign for Torver Commons and continue up a grassy track until you reach Kelly Hall Tarn. This is a pretty little tarn with fabulous views across to the Old Man of Coniston and Dow Crag, on your left. Follow the track which goes left around the tarn, and then passes a small rocky buttress. Proceed along the path until the landscape opens out. Ahead of you, on your right, is Long Moss Tarn.

2. As you reach an angle in the stone wall, go straight ahead, keeping the end of the tarn on your right. The track ascends for a short distance but is indistinct. You now reach the highpoint of the walk. On your right is Coniston Water; to your left are the mountains of the Old Man of Coniston, Swirl How and Wetherlam. Continue down the path.

3. Your route makes another short ascent before starting to descend

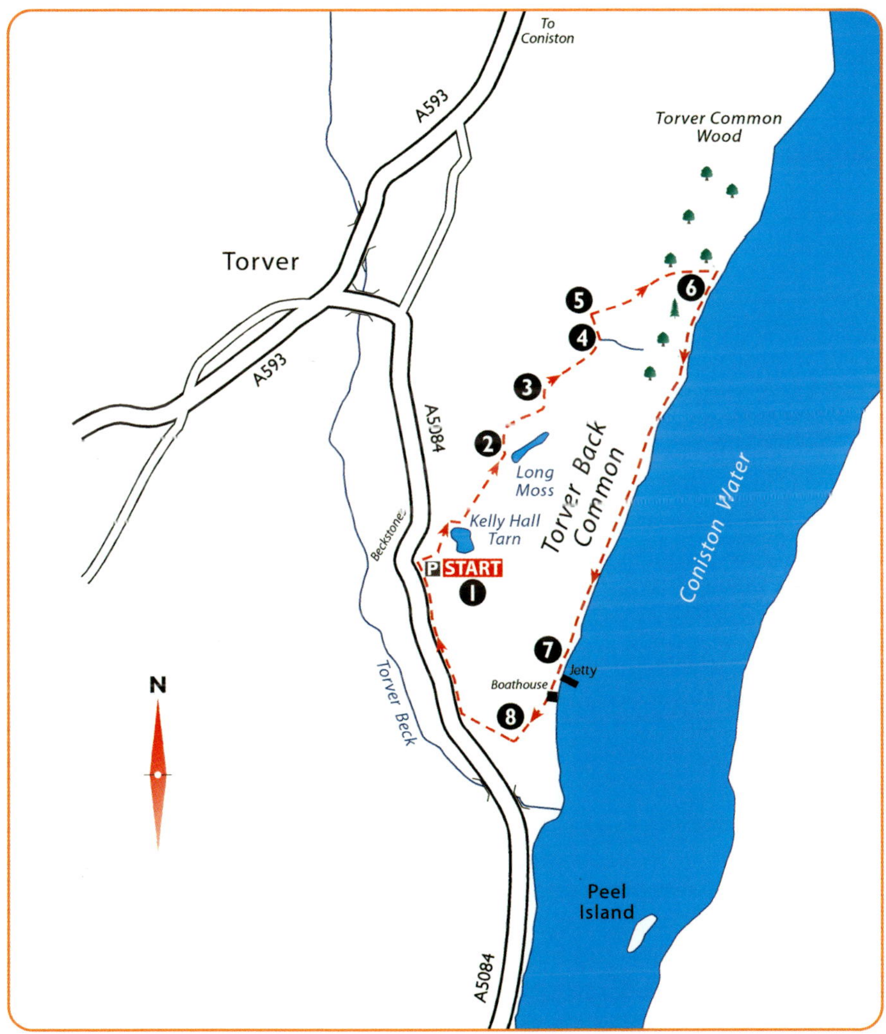

again along a faint track. There is a stone wall on your left, about 30 metres away. Ignore a path that bears left and goes into woodland through a wooden gate which is marked private. Carry on, keeping the wood over to your left. The path is occasionally indistinct.

4. You will pass through an area of gorse bushes and bracken on a narrow path. Soon afterwards you will approach a small stream with a large holly tree beside it. The path forks just before you get to the stream.

Ignore the path which bears right and heads down the valley following the stream. Take the path on the left, cross the stream, and then ascend beside a stone wall on your left. As you reach the end of this section of wall, continue ahead, following the most obvious path, which heads towards a clump of silver birch trees.

5. Before you reach the silver birch trees you will arrive at a T-junction in the path. Go left here, towards the birch trees, and then descend into a small valley. When you reach another junction in the path, go right and follow the obvious, rocky path, which descends through pleasant woodland towards the lake. Continue until you reach the lake shore. Go right here, along the shoreline, following the fingerpost marked 'public footpath Sunnybank'; Coniston Water will be on your left.

6. Follow the lake-shore path through woodland. There are several places along the shore that make ideal picnic spots. Go through a wooden gate into mixed woodland; then proceed through another gate and continue across a small stream. You will eventually emerge from the woods onto a rocky path, edged with gorse and bracken. Continue following the path as it sticks to the shoreline.

7. You will pass a wooden bench beside the lake and then reach Sunnybank jetty, which is used by the Coniston passenger launch. Across to your left is Peel Island. This is the stretch of water where Donald Campbell made his final run.

8. Your route now bears right, leaving the lake shore and ascending the hillside beside a stone wall. You will shortly reach a faint branch in the path. Bear right here and head up the rising grassy track. Keep on until you reach the road. Go right here, and continue until you reach your starting point. Take extra care on this section of road.

NEARBY ATTRACTIONS

The town of Coniston is a popular tourist destination and is the location of the **Ruskin Museum**. The 400-year-old **Black Bull** in Coniston (telephone: 015394 41335) is the perfect place to enjoy a pint of the award-winning Bluebird Bitter, which is brewed behind the pub. You can obtain more information about the area from Coniston Tourist Information Centre, Ruskin Avenue, Coniston, LA21 8EH, telephone: 015394 41533.

WINDERMERE FROM BOWNESS-ON-WINDERMERE

This walk incorporates short ferry crossings to reach the other side of the lake and to make your return. There are good views across Lake Windermere and its largest island, Belle Isle. Your route includes a short, energetic climb up through Station Scar Wood.

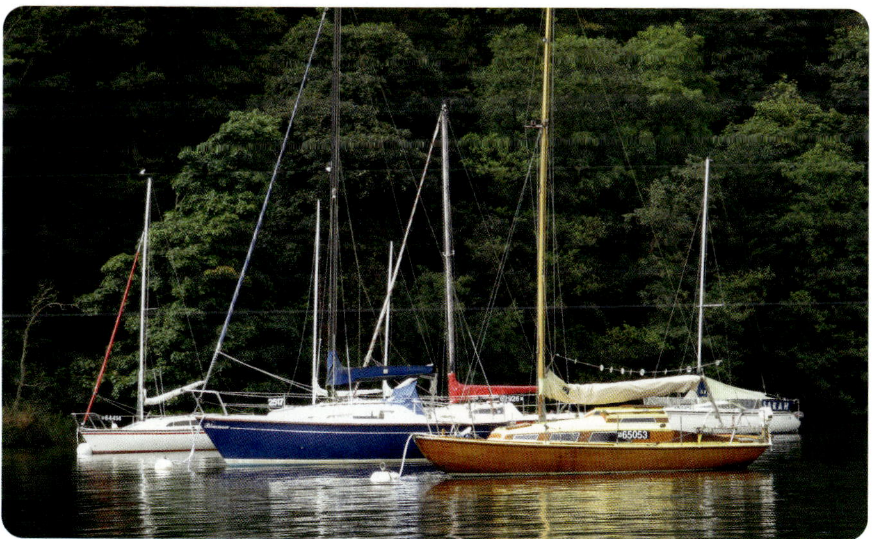

The popular Lake Windermere

- **HOW TO GET THERE:** Bowness-on-Windermere is located on the eastern shore of Lake Windermere. Windermere Quays Visitor Centre is in Glebe Road, just off the A592, to the left (as you face the lake) of the piers where boat trips depart.
- **PARKING:** The pay-and-display car park opposite the visitor centre.
- **LENGTH OF THE WALK:** 3.9 miles/6.3 kilometres. **MAP:** OS Explorer Map OL7 (GR SD 398965).
- **TERRAIN:** There is a tough little ascent up through the woods on the other side of the lake, and then a steady descent to the lake shore. The remainder of the route is level and easy to follow.

Bowness-on-Windermere developed after the opening of the railway line from Oxenholme and Kendal to Windermere in 1847. It became a popular Victorian resort and, in the late 19th century, wealthy businessmen from Lancashire built large mansions overlooking the lake. Arthur Ransome based the lakeside town of Rio in his book *Swallows and Amazons* on Bowness. Many of the impressive Victorian residences have now been converted to hotels, and today Bowness-on-Windermere is Cumbria's most popular destination.

Lake Windermere is the largest natural lake in England. It is 10.5 miles long and stretches from Ambleside to Newby Bridge. It reaches almost one mile wide at Millerground and has a maximum depth of 210 feet near its northern end. The name Windermere is derived from the Old Scandinavian name *Vinandr* and Old English mere 'lake', and the lake was known as *Winander Mere* or *Winandermere* until the 19th century.

Belle Isle, the largest island in the lake, is visible from your walk. It is one mile long and was once home to the Roman commander of Ambleside, who built a villa here. An unusual circular house, which dates from 1774, now stands on the island.

THE WALK

1. From the car park, join the pavement beside Glebe Road and then go left. Soon the road bends to the left and you will see a wooden fingerpost on the opposite side of the road, pointing down a track under some trees. Leave the road here and follow this track. After approximately 50 metres, go through the metal kissing gate on your left into Cockshott Point. Follow the main track. To your right is Lake Windermere. Belle Isle, with its dome-topped building, is visible across the water. Proceed along the path, following the edge of the lake round a bay that provides shelter for dozens of boats.

2. At the next metal kissing gate, go right. Proceed through a small wooded area which leads to a boatyard. A small café is located on the right. Keep straight on, and then through the gap in the stone wall, which takes you onto the road. Go right here, following the wooden fingerpost which directs you to 'Hawkshead via ferry'. Follow the road until you reach the ferry point. A cable-operated car and pedestrian ferry operates from the slipway. The price at the time of writing is 50 pence for pedestrians.

3. Take the ferry across to the opposite shore.

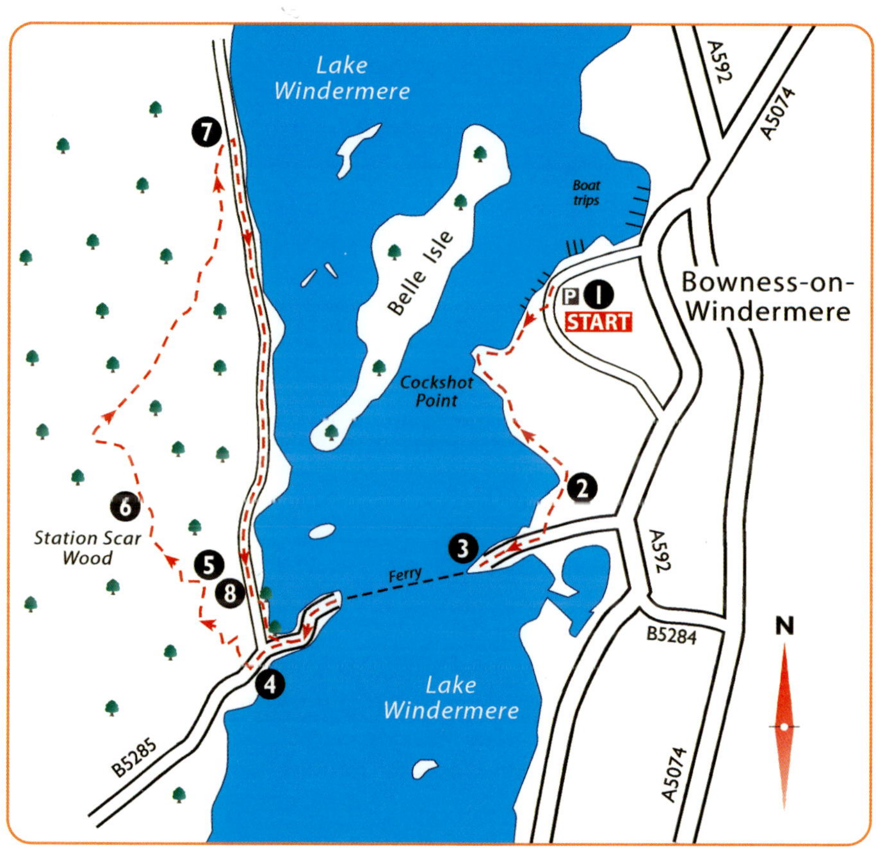

Windermere ferry has been operating for more than 500 years. The original ferry was made of wood and was rowed across the lake. The Mallard is diesel-powered and carries up to 18 cars – it is the only ferry in the Lake District that takes cars – and over 100 passengers. It takes ten minutes to cross Windermere from Ferry Nab, just south of Bowness, to Ferry House at Far Sawrey.

4. At the opposite side of the lake, follow the road. (Public toilets are available near the slipway.) The road bears left. Ignore the fingerpost pointing right, located just before the road bends to the right, and continue along the road. Once you pass a road junction on your right (to the 'lake shore and Harrowslack'), watch out for the fingerpost on your right, which is situated a short distance from the junction. Follow this fingerpost, which reads: 'public footpath Hill Top via Sawrey, Ash

Landing and Claife Station'. This leads you off the road and up through woodland.

5. Ignore the footpath which descends left and keep ascending, following the wooden fingerpost: 'public footpath Claife, white post route'. You will reach Claife Station, which is owned by the National Trust. Continue climbing through the dense woodland. Stick to the main path. It is steep in parts. You will arrive at a small plateau, a good place to rest for a while. The path now bears right, following a fence. Proceed along the path, and cross a rocky slab, which needs a little extra care in wet conditions, as it can be slippery. Carry on along the undulating path.

6. Stick to the main path as you make your way through the wood. After a straight section, with a stone wall on the right and a fence on the left, you will reach a wooden kissing gate and a T-junction in the path. Turn right and follow the white-topped fingerpost signed 'bridleway lake shore'. Go through a wooden gate and enter more woodland. Your route now descends towards the lake shore. Keep to the main path.

7. As you approach the lake, bear right and go over the stile and head towards the lake shore. When you reach the lakeside road, turn right and follow the road. This leads you back towards the ferry point. As you walk along, there are good views across the lake on your left. Carry on down the road, passing a National Trust car park on your right. You will see more boats in the bay to your left.

8. Look for a fingerpost on your left, inscribed 'public footpath to ferry'. Turn left here and leave the road. Follow the footpath through a wooded area that fringes the lake. You will pass buildings on your right and then emerge through double wooden gates onto the road. Go left here and follow the road a short distance to the ferry point where you alighted earlier. After re-crossing the lake by ferry, return to Bowness-on-Windermere by your original route.

NEARBY ATTRACTION

Bowness-on-Windermere is a very popular tourist town with good facilities. Windermere Lake Cruises run enjoyable cruises round the lake. More information is available from Bowness-on-Windermere Tourist Information Centre, Glebe Road, Bowness-on-Windermere, LA23 3HJ, telephone: 01539 442895.

RIVER KENT FROM STAVELEY

This walk starts from St Margaret's Tower and follows a picturesque salmon river, the River Kent, through farmland and a charming little wood at Beckmickle Ing. En route, you pass two dramatic weirs and the site of an old mill. Wild flowers adorn the riverbank in season and the area provides a safe haven for a variety of wildlife.

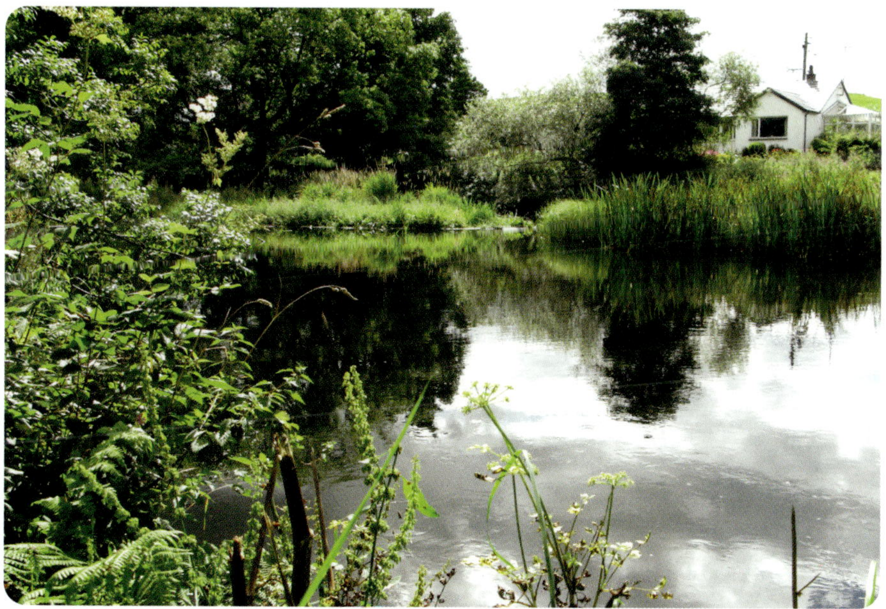

The mill pond above Bowston Weir

- **HOW TO GET THERE:** From Kendal follow the A591 towards Windermere. Follow the signs for Staveley, which lead you off the A591 and into the village. St Margaret's Tower is located in the centre of the village, next to the Duke William pub.
- **PARKING:** Road-side parking is available in various parts of the village.
- **LENGTH OF THE WALK:** 4.5 miles/7.25 kilometres. **MAP:** OS Explorer OL7 (GR SD 471981).
- **TERRAIN:** The route is mainly level.

The village of Staveley got its name from the woodworking industry that thrived in the area. *Staveley* is from Middle English *stave* 'stave, staff' and *leye* 'clearing, pasture'. Wood came from the forests that originally covered the surrounding hills, and the two rivers that flow through the village powered the mills that were used to process the wood.

Your walk starts from St Margaret's Tower, formerly a chapel which was built in 1388 on land given by Sir William de Thweng, Baron of Kendal and Lord of the Manor of Staveley. The chapel yard was the site of a protest in 1621 against James I's decision to claim land held by local tenants through the ancient border service rights. Tenants gathered outside the chapel to protest. Over 100 people were later indicted for forming part of the 'riotous meeting in Staveley chapel'.

Most of the route follows the River Kent. The River Kent is a salmon river, with fish typically between 4 to 8 lbs in weight, although in recent years catch returns have shown fish being taken up to 20 lbs. English Nature has designated the river as a Site of Special Scientific Interest, as the river supports the white clawed crayfish and white pearl mussel.

En route you will pass the site of the former Cowan Head Mill. A fulling mill, where cloth was cleaned and thickened, stood at Cowan Head in 1735. In 1746, it was converted to make paper, and in 1845 the paper manufacturer James Cropper leased Cowan Head Mill, subsequently buying it in 1854. Tragedy struck in 1893 when the chimney blew down, killing three workers.

THE WALK

1. Take the footpath that runs between the Duke William pub and St Margaret's Tower. Proceed down the path until you reach a wooden footbridge over the River Kent. Cross the bridge and then turn right, walking parallel to the river for a short distance. At a junction in the path, ignore the left turning which follows the wall. Instead, carry on through a kissing gate and up through a field.

2. Continue along the path, walking between two barns. A small yellow footpath badge is located on the barn on the right. Carry on along the track and then go through a wooded area. You will come to a wooden gate leading into a field. Beyond the gate there is a faint junction in the track; bear left here and pass a large boulder beside a small tarn. Proceed through a boggy section of field.

3. Continue alongside the large hawthorns which mark the edge of an

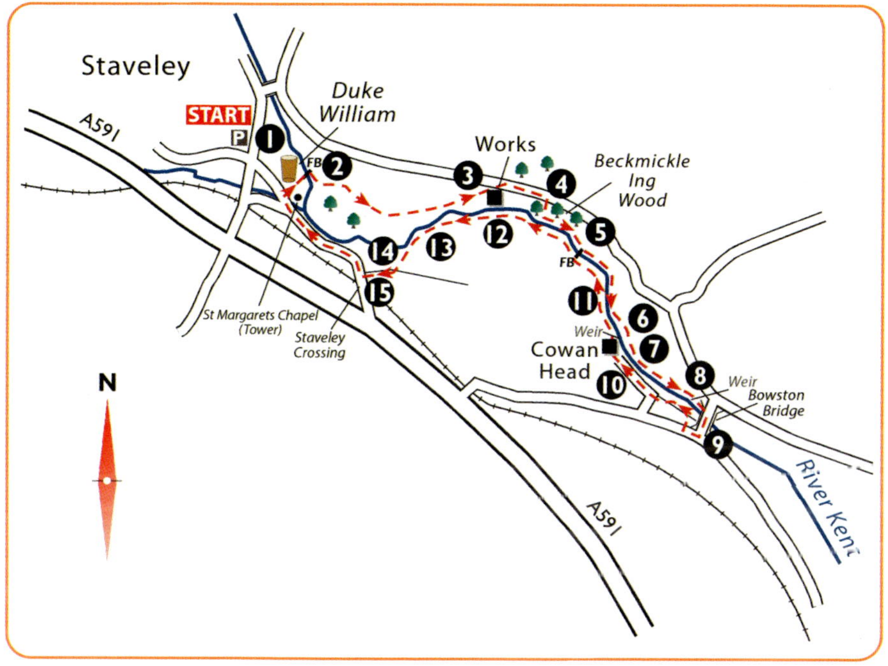

old field boundary, and then pass the end of a stone wall. Climb the five-step stile, which takes you over a stone wall and into another field. Go over the next stile, beside a wooden gate, and then across a tiny stream. Continue until you reach a kissing gate beside a wooden gate. Go through the gate and then onto the road. Turn right here and follow the road past the water treatment plant.

4. You will soon reach Beckmickle Ing, a pretty wood owned by the Woodland Trust. Leave the road at this point and descend through the wood on the path. Once you reach the river bank, go left, following the path through the woods, with the river on your right.

5. Cross the wooden footbridge over a small stream. Stick to the main path until you meet a major path which descends from your left. At this point turn right. Keep on until you arrive at a wooden stile over a fence. Climb the stile onto a farm track. To your right is a metal gate, with a bridge beyond it (no access). Go straight over the farm track and follow the public footpath sign through a kissing gate and into the next field. Keep to the edge of this field and walk roughly parallel to the river.

6. Go through the next kissing gate and along the edge of a golf course. Head towards the large white-painted buildings in front of you. The river widens here into a large mill pond. You will soon reach an impressive weir with a fish pass. This is the site of the former Cowan Head Mill.

7. From the weir, go uphill beside the stone wall and then under power lines. The path is very faint here. Keep close to the stone wall on your right. The path then starts to descend, passing an entrance to the Cowan Head complex. You will see a low post displaying a footpath badge, which directs you through the wooded area next to the river.

8. Continue following the path through farm fields, crossing several wooden stiles until you arrive at impressive Bowston weir, which looks like a mini Niagara Falls.

9. Continue downstream, through the field, keeping next to the fence. The river is now out of view on your right. At the end of the fence line you will reach a small stream. Go right, over a stile, and then go immediately left along a short track which leads to a road. Turn right here and follow the road over Bowston Bridge. You will reach a T-junction. Turn right here and follow the road. Once you have passed Kent Close on your right, turn right to leave the road and follow the fingerpost for Dales Way and Staveley .

10. Pass several cottages and Bowston weir mill pond, which you saw earlier from the opposite bank. Your route bears right as you pass a bungalow, and goes along a short section of track which then leads onto a road. Go right here and follow the road. Carry on past the Cowan Head complex and then through a group of attractive cottages.

11. Keep straight on. Go through a metal gate and then onto the river bank. This is an enchanting part of the river. Ahead of you is a large barn beside the bridge that you saw earlier from the opposite bank. Continue past the bridge and then the barn. Carry on over a stone step stile over the wall, and climb a rocky section of path overlooking the river. Go through a metal gate, and then through a field before crossing a high step-stile.

12. Continue through fields to a wide grassy area near the river. Climb into a wood over a high step-stile next to the river. Then turn immediately right, following the edge of a low stone wall. Cross another step stile. After emerging from the wood, make your way across an open field. Keep to the right and follow the river. Pass an old bed-head used as part of the fence.

13. Go through a metal gate into the next field, with a stone wall on your right. The river is out of view at this point. Follow the faint path across the field. Your route bends round to the right and leaves the field at the bottom right-hand corner. It then continues along a farm track that runs between two stone walls. The river now comes into view again on your right.

14. You will reach a wooden gate and a kissing gate. A sign on the gate reads 'Please keep to the public footpath'. Just beyond the gate, the river bends away to the right, and you will reach a fork in the path. At the fork, bear left and go through the kissing gate next to the metal gate which displays a hand-painted sign: 'footpath to Staveley'. Then follow the Dales Way fingerpost and trace the path through the field.

15. You will reach another gate and kissing gate. Once through the gate, go right, following the Dales Way fingerpost. Continue until you meet the main road. Turn right here and head towards Staveley. You will pass Stock Bridge Farm, which dates from 1638. Keep straight on, passing the Eagle and Child pub, and carry on over the road bridge across the River Gowan. You will soon reach the centre of the village and your starting point.

NEARBY ATTRACTION

The **Mill Yard** in Staveley, located behind the Duke William pub, includes a varied selection of retail and industrial businesses, including a café, a bakery, a brewery, and the UK's largest bike shop. It also contains furniture workshops and artists' studios and galleries. The **Eagle and Child**, Staveley, telephone: 01539 821320.

HODBARROW LAGOON FROM HAVERIGG

This route makes its way around Hodbarrow Lagoon and along the top of the Outer Barrier, with the sea to your left and the lagoon on your right. You will pass the ruins of a former windmill, as well as a recently restored lighthouse which dates from 1905. Take binoculars to get close-up views of the many species of birds that live on the lagoon and common seals, which from the sea wall can often be seen basking on the sandbanks.

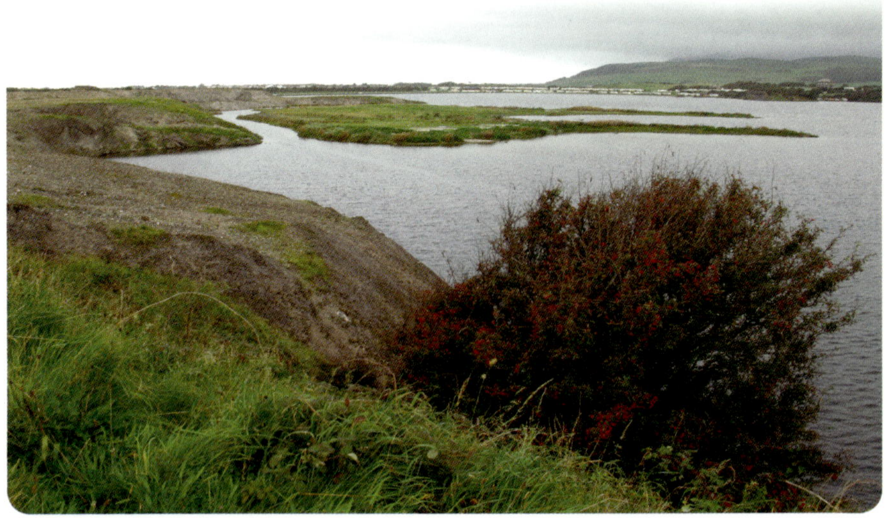

Hodbarrow Lagoon

- **HOW TO GET THERE:** From the A595, follow the A5093 to Millom. From there follow signs to Haverigg.
- **PARKING:** The large car park next to the seashore in Haverigg (free of charge at the time of writing).
- **LENGTH OF THE WALK:** 4 miles/6.4 kilometres. **MAP:** OS Explorer OL6 (GR SD 159784).
- **TERRAIN:** Mainly flat and along obvious paths.

Haverigg lies on the Duddon estuary, a short distance from the town of Millom. It is a small seaside fishing and farming village, tucked away on the south Cumbria coast. Haverigg gets its name from the Old Scandinavian *hafri* 'oats' and Old English rigg 'ridge', and can be interpreted as 'ridge where oats are grown'.

Hodbarrow Reserve occupies the site of a former iron ore mine. Mining began here in the 1850s and continued until 1968, when the pit closed. In its heyday, the mine employed over 1,000 men and produced half a million tons of ore a year. A concrete barrier was built to keep out the sea at high tide. This was breached after a few years and was replaced by the outer barrier wall which you see today. The extensive lagoon was created when the pumps were turned off and the mine workings flooded.

The reserve is now a haven for wildlife, with twelve species of mammal and six species of reptiles and amphibians recorded, including the endangered natterjack toad. Nineteen species of butterflies, including the dark-green fritillary, are found here too. In spring and early summer the reserve is alive with birdsong. Whitethroats and sedge and willow warblers take up residence, having arrived from Africa. The little tern arrives in mid-April to nest here. In autumn the numbers of wading birds increases, and curlews, sandpipers, greenshanks and black-tailed godwits can be spotted in the reserve.

THE WALK

1. From the car park walk towards the village. Follow the pavement alongside the river inlet, keeping the river on your right. The inlet provides safe mooring for small boats. When you reach the road bridge over the river, turn right and cross it. Then turn right again and follow the narrow footpath that goes along the top of the river bank, towards the sea. A fingerpost and CCW sign direct the way.

2. Your route now bears left in front of boulders placed to protect the coastline. On your right is the harbour. Join a narrow, grassy track for a short distance. Pass a wooden marker post, and then, at a minor road, keep straight on, towards the gates of Port Haverigg Holiday Village.

3. Follow the left-hand fingerpost ('public byway Steel Green'), which is located just to the left of the gates. Your route runs parallel to the road within the holiday complex, and then joins the road for a while. Keep going until you approach a cluster of stone buildings at Steel Green.

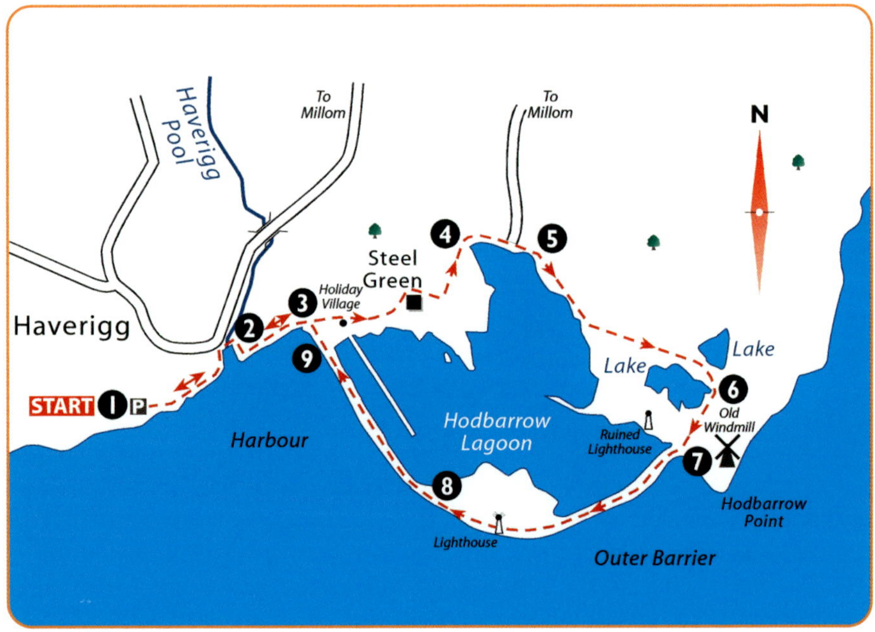

Here you will see a wooden fingerpost marked 'public byway'. Turn left and head towards the houses. The road initially bends left and then goes right, passing behind the houses. Ignore a footpath that goes left. Continue on a wide, tarmac path, passing through an avenue of trees.

4. You will reach a junction in front of the Commodore Hotel. Turn left here, along the minor road, keeping the hotel on your right. Continue down the minor road. Soon, another road joins your route from the left. Keep straight ahead. Follow the fingerpost indicating 'public byway Hodbarrow Point'. A short path, just to the right of the road, leads you beside the lagoon. You will reach a good viewpoint that overlooks the water. An information board tells you about the birds that live here. Carry on down the road.

5. Bear right when you reach the civic amenity site, and continue down a wide, rough track. On your left you will see a large information board giving details about Hodbarrow. Proceed down the track. Views of the lagoon are now blocked by trees. Keep to the main track. Your route veers away from the lagoon for a short distance, passing between two lakes, which for most of the year are hidden by foliage.

90

6. When you emerge from the tree-lined path you arrive at a bend in the main track. Bear right here and stick to the major track. On your right you will now see one of the lakes, which is surrounded by small cliffs. Proceed along the broad, gravel track.

Over to your right are the ruins of an old lighthouse, and those of a windmill become visible on the hillside on your left.

Carry on until you reach the sea. In front of you is an attractive sandy bay. An information board located here tells you about the Duddon estuary.

7. The broad track now bends to the right and follows a level, easy path along the top of the Outer Barrier.

There are excellent views across the sea on your left and the lagoon on your right. This is the perfect place to see some of the many species of birds that make the lagoon their home.

Carry on until you come to an attractive lighthouse, surrounded by benches. This is Hodbarrow lighthouse, built in 1905 to replace an older lighthouse and later refurbished following support from a local school.

8. As you approach Haverigg, on your left you will see part of the lovely sandy beach that lies along the coast at Haverigg. To your right is a corner of the lagoon which is used as a boating area by the holiday park. Continue along the top of the barrier.

9. When you reach the end of the path along the barrier you will meet a minor road. Go left here. Continue through the gates of the holiday park, which you passed at the beginning of your walk. From here reverse your footsteps to return to the starting point.

NEARBY ATTRACTIONS

Millom Folk Museum is open from Good Friday until 31st October each year. The **Punchbowl**, The Green, Millom (telephone: 01229 772605), sells the locally brewed, award-winning Beckstones beers.

RUSLAND POOL AND RIVER LEVEN FROM HAVERTHWAITE

This walk is a well-kept secret. The footpaths along Rusland Pool and the River Leven are often overlooked in favour of the more popular walking areas nearby; it is the perfect place to find solitude. Your walk follows two lovely rivers through farmland on level paths and along country lanes.

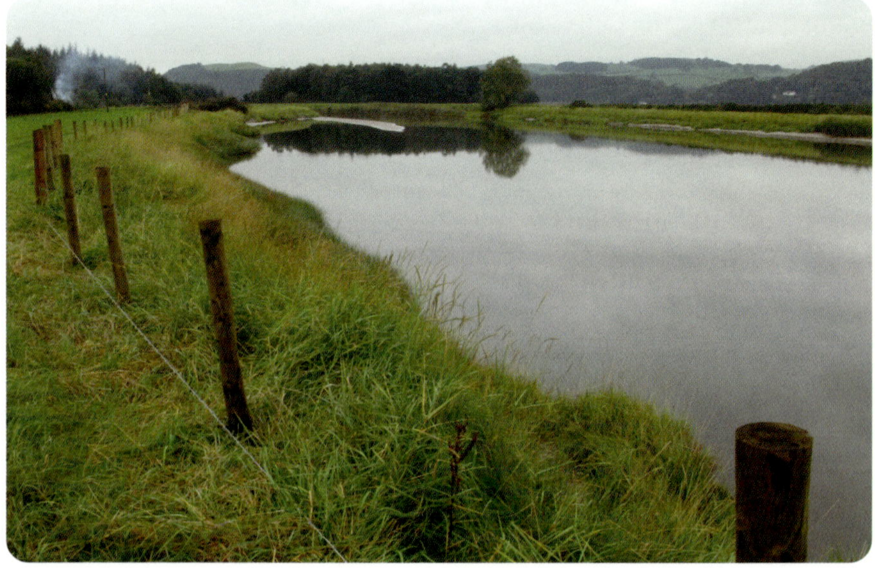

The River Leven

- **HOW TO GET THERE:** From the A590 follow the signs for Haverthwaite until you reach the Anglers Arms.
- **PARKING:** Limited roadside parking is available on Old Barrow Road that runs down the side of the pub.
- **LENGTH OF THE WALK:** 4.7 miles/7.6 kilometres. Map: OS Explorer OL7 (GR SD 347840).
- **TERRAIN:** Mostly flat, along easy paths. Some sections can be a little boggy after wet weather.

The River Leven drains Windermere from its southernmost point and flows for approximately eight miles into the northern reaches of Morecambe Bay. The river has one significant tributary, Rusland Pool, which drains Grizedale Forest and the Rusland Valley. Rusland Pool hasn't always been known by this name; it was known as the River Fosse in the 1500s.

In October 1794, Samuel Fell of Backbarrow was fishing for salmon when he saw a huge fish in the Leven. He cast his fly at the fish and hooked its back. He fought with the fish for over two hours until he managed to grab its tail and drag it onto the bank. He took his prize in a wheelbarrow to Haverthwaite, where the villagers gathered to see his catch: a 9 ft, 87 lb sturgeon. The next day he took the fish to Kendal market, where he sold it for ten pence per pound. Today, there are no sturgeon to be found in UK rivers, but the Leven continues to be a popular salmon river. At spawning time the fish can be seen jumping up the waterfalls at Backbarrow.

Your route crosses an old railway bridge over the River Leven, once the crossing point for the Furness railway line. The line was originally used to transport minerals but was later converted into a tourist line, which helped to develop the Lake District tourist industry. The line to Lakeside at the southern end of Lake Windermere lost its passenger service in 1965, but part of the line continues to operate today as the Lakeside and Haverthwaite Railway.

THE WALK

1. Proceed down Old Barrow Road, away from the pub, until you reach a wooden gate which blocks the lane. Pass through the gate and continue along the lane. At the end you will reach a gate and metal kissing gate. Go through the gate and into a field. Follow the wall on your right for a short distance until you reach stone steps that lead you over the wall. Once on the other side, turn left to follow the narrow path beside the wall. A short section of brambles needs to be negotiated. The path soon descends to meet the side of the A590.

2. Cross over the A590 and turn left. Follow the road, walking along the grass verge and then along the pavement, until you reach a junction. Turn right here and follow the road, which is signed 'Bouth, Rusland and Grizedale'. You will pass a Second World War pillbox on your right. Continue until you reach the T-junction at Causeway End. Turn left

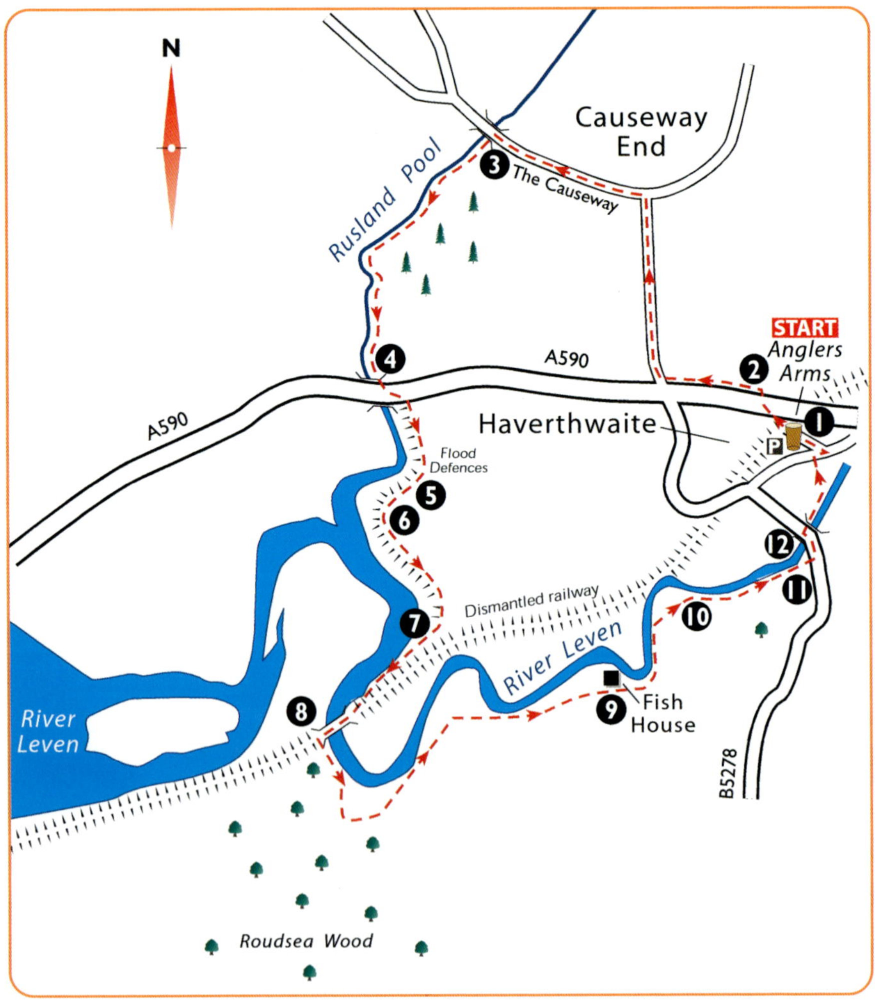

here and then follow the road until you reach the road bridge over
Rusland Pool.

3. Take the footpath on your left, immediately before the bridge, and
join the riverbank. Walk downstream, with the river on your right. Your
route follows a faint path along the grassy riverbank.

4. As you approach the concrete road bridge over the A590, look out
for a step stile on your left; you need to pass through a gap in the fence

94

on your left to get to it. Go over the stile and then through the wooden gate ahead of you. Ascend a series of steps up the roadside embankment, which take you onto the side of the A590, next to the bridge. Head straight across the road. Follow the path as it descends the roadside embankment and then bears right to meet a small stile. Cross over the stile and follow the path that traces the grassy top of the flood defence embankment.

5. You will pass a tall white post which marks the position of an underground gas line. Ignore the high step stile and footpath on your left and continue straight on, following the top of the flood defence embankment.

6. Rusland Pool now joins the much bigger River Leven. There are impressive open views across the river junction. Bear left here and follow the River Leven upstream, with the river on your right. The surrounding area is part of a sporting estate so you should stick to the footpaths and keep dogs on leads. Go through a wooden gate and then continue along the path.

7. Carry on until you reach a gate.

In front of you is a junction in the path. This is the site of the dismantled Furness railway line. The lines have been removed but you can still see their course.

Immediately before this junction, turn right at the wooden gate on your right (which is often kept open) and head towards the river bank. You will pass under overhead power lines. As you approach the riverbank, turn left to follow the fence which runs parallel to the bank. You will have the river on your right. The old railway bridge which crosses the river should soon be visible. Continue to the end of this field; then turn right in front of a metal gate and head towards the bridge.

8. Cross over the bridge and then pass through a metal gate. Go ahead for just a few metres, until you reach a small rise (the flood embankment). Turn left here into a wooded area, following the narrow path that runs along the top of the embankment. The river is now on your left. The route leaves the top of the embankment and winds through the trees. You will soon meet a minor road with a wooden fingerpost beside it. Turn left here and proceed along the road.

9. The road crosses the flood plain and the river is now out of view on your left. Mature oaks line this part of the route. As you progress you will pass a fisherman's hut beside the river on your left. Carry on. Passing a small derelict stone building on your left at Fish House, you will arrive at a point where the road widens. Immediately after this, look for a low wooden fingerpost that directs you left, off the road, over a small footbridge and then through a kissing gate. You now enter fields beside the river. Keep to the left and follow the river bank path.

10. At the end of the first field, go through a kissing gate and then over a footbridge across a tiny brook. Carry on. There are good views of the river at this point. At the end of the next field go through a wooden gate/kissing gate. After a few metres, you will reach a fork in the path. Stay left, keeping to the riverbank path.

11. Proceed through a third field and then through a kissing gate which takes you onto a minor road. Turn left here and follow the road until you reach a T-Junction with the B5278. Turn left, go along the B5278 and cross the stone road bridge.

12. Immediately after crossing the bridge, pass through a small gap on your right, just at the end of the bridge wall. A low wooden fingerpost (often hidden in foliage) directs you downstream, along the footpath beside the river, which is on your right. Continue along the riverbank path. You will reach a cluster of farm buildings. Go left here, passing between the houses, until you reach the road again. Turn right and follow the road. Carry on until you reach the Anglers Arms, and then turn left down Old Barrow Road back to your starting point.

NEARBY ATTRACTIONS

The **Lakeside and Haverthwaite Railway** runs traditional steam trains from the station at Haverthwaite (situated on the main A590), along the River Leven, to Lakeside at the southern end of Windermere. The **Lakes Aquarium** is also located at Lakeside. The **Anglers Arms**, Haverthwaite, telephone: 01539 531216.